Come Play!

Come Play!

The Craft of Movement and Games for Primary School

Author & Illustrator: Agnes de Souza
Cover Illustration: Laila Savolainen

Disclaimers

This book is designed to provide guidance and inspiration on the subjects discussed. It is not meant to, nor should it be used to diagnose or treat any developmental conditions. If you suspect your child has sensory integration challenges, please consult a specialist for a thorough assessment. Like all sporting activities, the games in this book may pose some inherent risk. Readers are advised to take full responsibility for their choice of games and equipment, and ensure the safety of the children in their care.

Every effort has been made to acknowledge the source of the games, but that is not always possible as many games have obscure origins and many variations. I am happy to receive feedback so that any omissions may be rectified.

In line with gender diversity, I have used the singular *they* as the pronoun of choice when gender identity is irrelevant to the game.

URL: http://www.movementthatmatters.com.au

Come Play! The Craft of Movement and Games for Primary School

Author and Illustrator: Agnes de Souza

Publisher: Movement That Matters, Fremantle, Western Australia

First published 2021

Interior and Cover Layout: Pickawoowoo Publishing Group

Print and Distribution: Lightning Source and Ingram

ISBN 978-0-6451333-0-1 paperback

ISBN 978-0-6451333-1-8 epub

ISBN 978-0-6451333-2-5 hardback

NATIONAL LIBRARY OF AUSTRALIA

A catalogue record for this book is available from the National Library of Australia

'Children's Games' by Pieter Bruegel the Elder (1560) oil on panel, is reproduced here with permission from KHM-Museumsverband.

'Fire and Ice' adapted from 'Games Children Play' by Kim Brooking Payne, published by Hawthorn Press. Reproduced with permission of the Licensor through PLSclear.

"Children learn with their bodies before they learn with their brains. Physical and sensory feedback derived from interaction with the physical world help to build the neural pathways necessary to form mental images of the world."

— **Sally Goddard Blythe**, *author of 'The Genius of Natural Childhood and What Babies and Children Really Need.*

Contents

Foreword

'Come Play! The Craft of Movement and Games for Primary School' is a much-needed book in times of pervasive bodily stasis and manic media consumption. Combining the latest scientific research with practices derived from Waldorf Education and the Waldorf inspired Extra Lesson, Agnes de Souza makes an eloquent case for an informed integration of intelligent play into the curriculum.

Starting with Sensory Integration Activities that form the foundation of hand-heart-head connection, the book offers valuable insights into why movement and games are so uniquely important.

What will make this book particularly appealing to parents, carers, therapists, Kindergarten teachers and teachers is its age-appropriate structure. de Souza not only suggests a great variety of games for each age group, but introduces them in a threefold manner, firstly by describing the developmental stage of the child. Secondly, she explains why certain movements and games are salutary for a particular phase of childhood and lastly, what stance and attitude will serve the teacher best. This makes 'Come Play!' an immensely practical and easy to use manual for anyone seeking inspiration on how to engage the whole child in meaningful and healthy ways.

Written by an expert teacher and therapist, 'Come Play!' is a book that anybody working with children will undoubtedly benefit from.

Horst Kornberger
Educator, Writer, Speaker and Interdisciplinary Artist

Preface

The idea for this book came from a colleague who was intrigued with my movement programme. She saw that something about those sessions met the children's needs; that they enjoyed, looked forward to, and were fully engaged during my sessions. She would ask for activities she could use in her class, whether for fun or for remediation. She was time poor and asked me to recommend a book.

My movement classes draw heavily on my experience as an Extra Lesson® and Bothmer® Gymnastics Teacher. I have a grounding in child development, a foundation in anthroposophy, and a toolbox of movement activities and games acquired from years of training and learning from books and conferences, gems from colleagues, and those I made up or adapted, as well as games my students taught me. A book that covers it all? Impossible! No single book can cover everything, but perhaps I could share my approach!

The book idea took hold, a seed was planted, and this is the result! In this book, I present movement activities and games imbued with joy, enlivened with imagination and informed by child development and pedagogy.

My work has been inspired by the idea that the teaching activity should be filled with 'living artistry'[1]; and that while a healthy development depends much on nature or heredity, it reaches its fullest potential with conscious education, along with games, play, storytelling and imagery as allies.

---

[1] (Down, 2012)

Come Play!

The games and activities presented here are guides and inspiration, not recipes. We all have our favourites, and many here are adapted to my teaching style, the circumstances under which I taught, the equipment, or lack thereof, as well as the differing needs of children. If a game does not resonate with you, don't use it. If a story does not resonate with you, create your own.

Acknowledgments

My own teaching has been enhanced by watching great teachers teach. I would like to thank Dan Freeman, my teacher and mentor, for years of training, and for instilling in me a love of Bothmer Gymnastics and playing games, and for the opportunity of watching him teach in school. My thanks also to Martin Baker and the team at Michael Hall Steiner School for allowing me to observe them teach, and to Bothmer Movement International (BMI in UK and Hungary) for summer intensives, with amazing teachers and games galore.

Games come alive with the people you play with, and I light up just thinking about my Bothmer Gymnastics colleagues who have shared the journey of movement and games with me. Thank you for years of games and comradery, sweat and tears, insight and inspiration, laughter and debate, shared meals and dormitories, and support and empathy with injuries and broken toes.

I thank my students, who have gifted me with their trust, openness, joy and enthusiasm. I have learnt so much just playing with you.

My heartfelt gratitude to Louise Swanson, a dear friend and Bothmer Gymnastics colleague, who stood steadfastly by me on this writing journey, and for generously sharing her insight and wisdom. I am indebted to Sean Burke and Titus Witsenburg, for their constructive criticism and invaluable insight, and to Horst Kornberger for writing the Foreword to my book. Thank you to Karen Peradon-Alaga, my copy editor for her friendship, guidance and support.

Come Play!

I am grateful to my family for the gift of time and space to write this book, for playing the games with me, and for their technical and emotional support throughout this writing and publishing process.

Together, they held me and helped shaped this book.

How to use this Book?

Chapter One provides a brief theoretical perspective of 'why' and 'how' movement is important. It may appeal to all who care for or work with children, to know how movement grows the child, and how to spot the tell-tale signs of motor development difficulties and how they relate to learning challenges.

Chapter Two contains motor development and sensory integration exercises that could be included into the parent, teacher, educator, camp facilitator or therapist's toolkit. They are but a window into the world of sensory integration and do not replace professional therapy.

In Chapter Three, I discuss games and their importance, and provide suggestions on presenting, managing and creating your own games. This may be useful for the class teacher, games teacher, novice teacher or anyone interested in playing games with children.

Chapter Four covers age appropriate games for the primary years, from One to Six (ages 7 to 12). The year level indicated assumes that the first primary school year begins the year the child turns seven. This is not necessary the case in some countries, and if that is so for you, please use the age indicated as a guide.

Each year level begins with a developmental picture of the child, the movement emphasis, and the teacher's 'sheath of authority' for that year and age. They are given as guides, not dogma, based on my best understanding of the pedagogy that supports them, and can be played from that age or year level onwards (even adults have been known to enjoy these games!). This information may be helpful for the class or physical education teacher, parent, camp or games facilitator or anyone interested in the value of games. The stories for each of the games are my own, except otherwise acknowledged.

A suggested list of songs and verses can be found in the Appendix.

Chapter 1

Movement, Play, Games and Sports

Movement activities, play, games and sport. What is the difference? Movement activities are games, actions or activities that encourage motor development and the building of gross and fine motor coordination.

Play, in its purest form is unstructured physical activity. Children climbing trees, playing with their dolls, or making mud pies are play activities.

Games are playful activities involving more than one person. It has a minimal set of rules, some equipment and coaching, and may be cooperative or competitive. Hide and seek, tag and storm the castle are games involving some strategy, running and chasing.

Sport is a structured form of physical activity, pertaining to an individual's skills and performance. They can be recreational or competitive, with teams, coaches and the keeping of scores. Basketball, rugby, soccer and volleyball are such examples.

This book is about movement activities and games: movement activities that nurture growing bodies, and games that are age appropriate and meet the developmental needs of the growing child.

Why is Movement important?

The body is the vehicle through which we express ourselves, in movement, gestures, stance or speech. Movement is more than just the moving of bones, joints and muscles. When one part moves, the body as a whole responds[2]; a seamless integration of a living body, with many systems working in harmony.

The Human Body was Designed for Moving

From an anatomical perspective, the human body was designed for moving. The average human musculoskeletal system is made up of 206 bones, 360 joints (point of attachment between two bones) over 600 muscles, three types of cartilage (soft, gel like padding between bones that protect joints and aid movement), over 4000 tendons (tissues connecting muscle to bone), 900 ligaments (tissues connecting bone to bone) and other connective tissues.

Our skeletal muscles, all 639 of them, are like a kind of elastic tissue, working in pairs to move body parts by pulling on the bones they are attached to. One in a pair pulls (contracts) to move a bone or bend a joint while the other relaxes, and then they reverse roles to bring the muscle back to its original position.

Together, the muscular and skeletal systems work to move the body as well as provide form and support for the organs. Healthy muscles drive human movement, and movement in turn lubricates the body and preserves muscle quality. Lack of quality movement affects joint mobility, causing stiffness, limited range of motion and joint degeneration, further limiting movement. In other words, we use it or we lose it.

---

[2] (Myers, 2014)

The Neuromuscular System

Muscles may consist of thousands, or tens of thousands, of small muscle fibres, and a muscle's strength depends mainly on how many fibres are present. Specialised fibres, called muscle spindles, found in the belly of muscles, act as proprioceptors, as they register muscle lengthening and the rate of the change in muscle length.

There are over six trillion muscle fibres in the human body, each commanded by one of the seven trillion nerves that transmit signals between the brain, spinal cord, and the rest of the body. They control the skeletal muscles, interpret sensory information, and coordinate the activities of the body.

The Brain

The brain is like the master controller. It responds to stimulation from the environment by creating neural pathways to develop new skills and abilities. Within the cortex of the brain are billions of tiny nerve cells that connect and communicate with other cells throughout the body, in a complicated network. These cells continue to develop, adapt and modify its neural connections to grow new brain cells.

The Muscle and Brain Connection

Neuroscientific evidence show that the same areas of the brain are activated when learning as when moving[3]. Every movement the body makes, whether it is learning to crawl, walk or write, learning a new language or playing an instrument, provides sensory information for the brain to process, adapt to and form new neural pathways, which in turn enhances cognitive functioning.

The brain's ability to change and grow stronger the more we use it, has led to the brain being compared to a muscle – the more you use it, the stronger it gets.

---

[3] (Jensen, 2005) (Playground Professional, 2015)

Movement and Development

Many studies have linked movement to child development and learning, in areas such as memory, perception, language, attention, behaviour emotion and decision making[4].

Rudolf Steiner[5] the originator of Waldorf Education, names the three major developmental milestones in early childhood as walking, speaking and thinking. The process goes in two ways, according to the principles of cephalo-caudal (from head to foot) and proximo-distal (centre to periphery, i.e. the fingers and toes).

From head to foot, the young child learns to master an array of movement patterns, initially unskilled and uncoordinated, towards a gradual control of their muscles in order to focus their eyes, lift their head, grasp objects, crawl, sit, stand, balance and then walk.

Their fine motor control develops from the centre out, from the gross towards dexterity of fingers and toes. This also includes the subtle development of the speech mechanism from the larynx to the lips, which culminates in speech.

Interwoven with motor development is sensory development, which also follows a foundational progression, beginning with awareness of the bodily kinaesthetic senses to the perceptual senses. A certain level of motor and sensory maturity is needed before the child is considered ready for formal learning in school.

---

[4] (Goddard, 2002)

[5] (Steiner, 1923)

The Sensory Integration System

We become aware of our world by way of sensations (detecting sensory information) and perception (the integration, interpretation and conscious experience of these sensations). We engage with the world when we act on this information through our movements.

Ayres[6] describes sensory integration as the organisation of sensations; of putting together all the senses that stream into the human body into a coherent experience. Imagine peeling and eating an orange, and all the sensory information coming through our eyes, nose, mouth, skin, fingers, muscles and joints, working together to bring us this experience of eating an orange.

Most of us are familiar with the five senses through which we process information: *touch, taste, sight, smell, hearing.* Modern science has expanded this list to include *proprioception* (the perception or awareness of the position and movement of the body), *vestibular* (balance and motion) and *interoception* (how our body tells our brain what is going on inside our body).

Yet, in 1909, Rudolf Steiner proposed a way of looking at human development through the spectrum of the twelve senses[7] (*touch, life, movement, balance, smell, taste, sight, warmth, hearing, language, thought,* and *ego)*. The first four senses relate to the physical or Willing aspect of the human being. They lay the foundation for all other senses, particularly the four higher or Thinking parts of the human being. Mediating between these two polarities are the middle senses that relate to the Feeling realm of the human being.

This pedagogy of educating the whole person through the Hands (Willing), Heart (Feeling) and Head (Thinking) has implications for education and is what guides much of the resources described in this book.

---

[6] (Ayres, 2007)

[7] (Steiner, 1916)

The Pedagogy of the Twelve Senses

These senses are 'helpers' of perception, helping us perceive and make meaningful our sensory experience. A sense does not just work on its own, but in concert with all other senses, and each is related to a polar opposite sense.

Hence while a movement curriculum works primarily through the physical senses, it affects all other senses, in particular the higher senses. In other words, to reach the thinking (Head), we need to work through the physical (Hands), with the feeling realm (Heart) acting as the bridge.

This view of the twelve senses has implications for teaching and gives insight to what is unfolding in a child's physical, cognitive, emotional and spiritual development. A healthy development of these senses contributes to a healthy development of the human being[8]. A healthy movement curriculum works strongly through the physical senses to influence the physical and higher order cognitive senses.

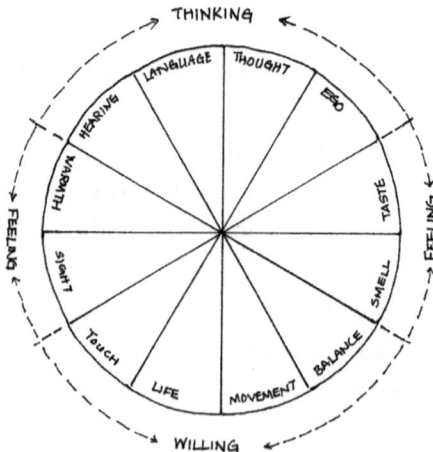

---

[8] (Soesman, 1990)

I. The Sense of Touch

The sense of Touch is the body's inner experience of contact with the environment. We experience ourselves inwardly by becoming aware of a boundary, a sense of where we begin and end, and where another person begins. The skin, the largest organ of the human body, is the organ for the sense of touch. Nerve endings below the skin relay messages to the brain to register a sensation.

Newborns are born with this capacity, and they learn about their environment through touching and feeling. The sense of Touch teaches the child where their boundaries are, and is a bridge connecting the individual to the outside world. It can be nurtured with loving and soothing connection or it can be distorted by abuse (physical, verbal or sexual) or neglect.

A healthy development gives a sense of security as well as the ability to understand fear. A balance has to be struck between the child experiencing fear and learning to overcome it, to sheltering the child from any form of fear whatsoever. The moral value of games allows children to experience this fear in a safe and secure way.

The opposite to the sense of Touch is the sense of Ego or the 'I' sense. A healthy sense of Touch gives us the ability to perceive the I of another person. This is especially important in social interaction and interpersonal relationships.

2. The Sense of Life (Wellbeing)

The organ for perceiving the sense of Life is the autonomous nervous system, (sympathetic and parasympathetic). It is attuned to all the movement and internal activities of the life body and is the body's sensation of well-being, our etheric life force. The sense of Life functions like a mirror of our internal activity[9]. We often take it for granted and only become aware of it when we are in physical discomfort.

This sense is functional at birth. When contented, the infant is peaceful and relaxed, feeling secure and comfortable. When in discomfort, the infant cries to alert their caregiver to their needs.

This sense is influenced by the rhythm and routine of our daily experience, of how we are cared for, loved, dressed, fed or nurtured. Developing this sense is about finding a balance between letting it flourish and mature totally protected and allowing the child to sense discomfort and pain.

The lesson from the sense of Life it that through pain and discomfort, we learn restraint. In movement and games, the child comes to be aware of their abilities and limitations. They learn to be patient, to take turns, to give and to receive.

The opposite to the sense of Life is the sense of Thought (concept), the ability to be open to another's point of view. How can one have empathy and compassion for another if one is closed to other viewpoints except our own?

---

[9] (Schoorel, 2004)

3. The Sense of Movement (Self-movement)

The sense of Movement is our ability to perceive our body's movements and posture. From the gross (walking, running) and the fine (sewing, writing) to the subtle (blink of an eye), we express ourselves through our bodies. The sense organ is in our muscles and the movement organisation, which include the muscle spindles, motor endplates, tendons and ligaments. When we move, even the smallest movement, our entire body is involved.

Muscular movement is the expression of nervous system activity. While children are born with this capacity to move, the organs of movement are not yet mature. Its maturity is co-dependent on that of the nervous system (a requirement for higher order thought processes), which is best effected by muscular movement.

Children thus grow through movement: crawling, walking, running and imitating the world around them, initially a little clumsy and uncoordinated, then with increasing intent and purpose. This is seen in the rhythm of moving from one activity to the next.

It is the inner movement, that of our intent or purpose that directs our outer movements. Limiting or distorting healthy movement affect us on a soul level, that of a sense of purpose. The ability to control our movements gives us a sense of freedom. A poor sense of movement is like a cramping of this freedom, a powerlessness.

In movement and games, children learn to use and coordinate their movements in space and time. This metamorphoses into a healthy sense of Language, the art of communication. Effective communication is more than mere words, it is an art and skill necessary for a successful living.

4. The Sense of Balance

The sense of Balance is how we relate to the world, and how we orient ourselves to the three-dimensional space around us to maintain our upright balance without falling over every time we move. The main organ of our balance (the vestibular system) is the ear, particularly the semi-circular canals in the inner ear, which are oriented at 90° to each other, thus in three dimensions of space. Sensors in our skin, joints and muscles also help us maintain our balance and coordination.

The spatial position of the young infant is horizontal. Through exercising the sense of movement and the maturation of the central nervous system, the child learns to hold their head up, sit up freely, pull themselves upright, walk, run, turn, move forward, backward and sideways. They learn to conquer gravity and space, and find a harmonious coexistence between the two to maintain balance.

On the soul level, our upright stance is our point of reference; how we are able express who we are as a person, and how we are then able to connect to the world.

In movement and games, the child learns to explore and conquer the space around them, learning to move freely in the three dimensions of space. Is it any wonder that the polar opposite of the sense of Balance is the sense of Hearing, the ability to be still in order to hear the intent behind the tones?

5. The Sense of Smell

The sense of Smell is how we attune to our environment, much of which happens on an unconsciousness level. It develops between the ages of three and nine, after which children are able to relate to the world of odours. Sensory receptors in our nose can distinguish at least one trillion different odours. Free nerve endings in the nasal mucosa have a short and direct route to parts of the brain involved in learning and memory.

This means that we can be influenced or swayed by smells because of their ability to conjure up memories. Smell is innately related to our instinct, judgment and drive. Like little radars, our noses 'sniff' things out. If something does not feel right, we sense or 'smell trouble' or 'smell a rat', or that something 'smells fishy', or simply that it 'stinks'.

To have a 'good nose' for something is to have the capacity of discernment, for what is morally right or wrong, for what is worthwhile and good. A scent, then, invokes judgment, and children quickly learn to trust their nose, sniffing out the inner qualities of people or situations.

Games foster the ability to trust our instincts, to judge the intent of the other, and also to fuel the drive to overcome obstacles. Games teach social and moral values. The polar opposite to the sense of Smell is the sense of Warmth, the capacity to radiate heartfelt warmth, interest, and connection to the world around us.

6. The Sense of Taste

The mouth is the beginning of the digestive process, so what we take in (physically or metaphorically) becomes us. Mucous membranes in the mouth begins this digestive process and chewing continues it to bring about the perception of taste, whether it is sweet or sour, bitter or salty, nourishing or otherwise.

On an emotional level, we take in something from the outer world, digest and perceive the 'inner side' of things. We can distinguish whether an experience is 'sweet' or has left us with a 'sour taste', or if we had to 'swallow a bitter pill'. To have 'good taste' is to have the ability to discern the inner quality of something or someone.

Our sense of Taste also informs our sense of Life. We know inwardly to seek food that comforts or heals, to distinguish the quality and care of food cooked with love, which in turn aids digestion on a physical and emotional level.

Infants are born with the ability to taste, and they can develop a healthy instinct for what to, and what not to eat. Our perception of Taste is further enhanced by our sense of Smell with sensory input from our nose, as well as from our sense of Touch.

Games and imagery in games allow for emotions, strategies and concepts to be digested in order to serve as a capacity for growth. The polar opposite to the sense of Taste, is the sense of Sight, the ability to discern the quality of a phenomenon.

7. The Sense of Sight

Through the eye, the world opens to us and we perceive the world as shapes, movement, distance, colour, proportions, depth, etc. We 'think' in our eyes to make sense of what we see, by adding what we expect to see to what we actually do see. In other words, our thoughts determine what we see. As a result, we have optical illusion, or an 'illusory insight'.

This sense connects us on an emotional, soul level to the outside world. We sense the mood of colours, how colours or the environment can sooth, calm or excite us. We may say 'what a sight to behold' or 'how depressing it looks'. A person with a 'good eye' is able to discern the inner quality of something, someone or phenomena.

The eye perceives images and colour and leaves us with a mental picture long after we have stopped seeing a particular image. When we try to remember a particular event that has occurred in the past, we usually see an image of the event.

We also say that a picture paints a thousand words, with the ability to give rise to imaginations or the capacity to come to imagination. Stories also create pictures in our mind's eye, thus enlivening imagination. Movement activities and games with imagery enlivens a child's soul.

The polar opposite of the sense of Sight is the sense of Taste, the ability to discern the inner quality of something or someone.

8. The Sense of Warmth

Through sensory nerve cells under our skin feeding back to the pineal gland, our sense of Warmth allows us to experience physical warmth as well as heartfelt warmth in our environment.

Like being bundled up snug and warm from the cold, having warm soup, hot cocoa or mulled wine, or being enveloped in a warm embrace and heartfelt connection with others in our community and environment creates warmth.

Curiosity leads us out into the world and if we are met with interest and warmth, our attention is held and sustained, and we are nourished. If we are met with a 'cold' shoulder, or are excluded, then we withdraw, hurt and alone.

The palms of the hands and the inside of the arms are more sensitive than the back of the hands or the outside of the arm. And we are more likely to trust and gravitate towards someone who offers us a 'warm handshake' rather than a cold one. Warmth is contagious, it radiates and connects all at once.

When children are met with warmth and interest in movement activities and games, they learn to develop their sense of Warmth. They become more capable of perceiving both physical warmth and cold, and in the metaphorical sense, the ability to deal with it.

The sense of Warmth enables one to trust our feelings for what may be. It relates to the sense of Smell, the ability for instincts, to discern what is morally right or wrong.

9. The Sense of Hearing

The ear is the sensory organ of both balance and hearing. The outer ear picks up sound waves (vibrations), the middle ear transfers sound waves into fluid-membrane waves and the inner ear converts them into neural impulses.

The nerve receptors for hearing are contained within the cochlear of the inner ear. These impulses travel to a relay station in the brainstem and then to the auditory cortex, the hearing part of the brain where they are converted into meaningful sound, or tone.

The sense of Hearing is both a social and internal activity. We cannot block our ears and they remain open, connected to the world. To consciously listen to another, to hear not just the content of the words, but the intent behind them, requires an inner stillness or quiet on our part.

In games, the ability to develop the sense of Hearing is enhanced by the developing of the sense of Balance, the ability to find our own uprightness. Children's movement exploration helps them conquer the three dimensions of space.

10. The Sense of Language (Word)

The sense of Language allows us to hear how tones form a language, even if we do not understand that particular language. In hearing, we take something of the external world into ourselves, and in the sense of language, we are processing the meaning behind what is expressed. We are trying to grasp how another communicates to us through the use of language.

The sense of Language is a potential that needs to be developed through exercise and exposure. The young child begins to perceive language and with the sense of movement, he begins to babble and then to speak the language in order to be connected to his environment.

In movement activities and games, children learn to communicate and negotiate. To understand another person's ideas, we must hear them expressed, and we express ourselves through our whole body. Thus language is not just heard by our ear, but by our whole musculoskeletal system.

The opposite to the sense of Language is the sense of Movement. When children develop their capacity for movement and coordination, they enhance their agility and flexibility, which then enhance the sense of Language.

II. The Sense of Thought (Concept)

The sense of Thought gives us the ability to understand and perceive the thoughts of others. It is the ability to be focused and open to another's viewpoint and to follow their line of reasoning.

The sense of Thought develops gradually from about 18 months. We learn to perceive the meaning behind a word or gesture, for if we do not perceive correctly, we cannot understand correctly.

To do so, one must put aside one's thoughts and concerns, or the images or concepts in one's mind, and try to give over to the other person's thoughts, to find out what they mean. Only then are we able to broaden our views and be able to bring it in connection with our own thoughts.

The sense of Thought is linked to its polar opposite, the sense of Life. Part of the sense of Life is focused on the body to observe bodily processes, and parts of it is focused on the mind to observe mental processes. When our nervous system is calm and relaxed, we are in a better position to engage, learn and create new neuropathways in the brain. In contrast, it is impossible to take in, retain or integrate new information when we are nervous or anxious[10].

A healthy sense of Life in childhood contributes to a healthy sense of Thought. When children participate in movement activities and games, they learn restraint as they experience the pain of losing, of taking turns and not monopolising the situation.

---

[10] (Lackner, 2016)

12. The Sense of Ego (I)

The sense of Ego or I, is how we connect to others in a true and meaningful way. It comes from within, through the sense of Touch. At the other end of the spectrum, the sense of another comes from the outside through the Ego sense, the ability to perceive and be sensitive to someone's individuality, or the Ego of another.

The sense of Ego perceives something that is not visible, the something that manifests as someone's essence. To truly meet and have a respectful interaction with another requires that we know our own boundaries, and the boundaries of the other.

Children develop this in an atmosphere of trust, when they are around others who set the example of discernment. Everything that a child experiences through touch prepares them for the Ego sense.

In games, children experience safety (within safe zones) and fear (when being chased in a tag game). They get to experience playing the chaser (the hungry shark or the mean farmer) as well as the chased (poor little sheep or rabbits). This gives them the opportunity to perceive a sense of the other.

The opposite to the sense of Ego is the sense of Touch, which acts like a bridge between perceiving and knowing our own boundary and that of another.

In Summary of the Twelve Senses

The paradigm of the twelve senses has been given as a guide, not as dogma. Burke[11] reminds us that what is more important than the actual number of senses, is that senses can be nurtured, be impaired or deteriorate. While we may distinguish them for deeper understanding, we need to remember that senses work together in a complex, interwoven and supporting manner. Having a rich firsthand sensory experience is still the young child's best teacher.

---

[11] (Burke, 2010)

What Affects Movement Development?

As a house needs a firm foundation, so too the human body. Interferences to early movement development is like having a house with faulty foundations upon which later development takes place. These developmental milestones create neural connections in the brain which lay the foundation for higher learning. Developmental delays are often the first signs that children may have learning difficulties later in life.

Reflexes

The infant is born with a cluster of involuntary or *primitive* reflexes, which are automatic movement patterns that respond to specific sensory stimulation. They develop in the womb and are present in the full-term baby. These allow the baby an active role in the birth process, to lay down essential survival skills, and provide the foundational patterns for later conscious control of movement.

Primitive reflexes are controlled by the lowest level of the brain: the spinal cord and the brain stem, and should be under voluntary control by the first year. Delays can contribute to academic, emotional and social challenges, and depending on the reflex that is retained, the child may be hypersensitive, startle easily, be fidgety, clumsy, anxious, or have trouble reading and writing.

Postural reflexes gradually replace primitive survival patterns to help the child gain subconscious control of posture, balance and motor coordination, a sign that the cerebellum, midbrain and cortex have matured sufficiently. These reflexes should be established when the child is about three and a half years old. An undeveloped postural reflex is like having an underdeveloped vocabulary, and this can affect learning and social adaptability. Tell-tale signs are poor balance, posture, coordination, bilateral integration and fine motor control.

Bilateral Integration

The two hemispheres of the brain are connected by a bundle of nerve fibres called the corpus callosum, which acts like a superhighway conduit for information sharing. The right hemisphere, responsible for the logical or analytical processing, controls the left side of the body. The left hemisphere controls the right side of the body and is involved in more creative processing, emotions and spatial orientation.

The ability to accurately perceive sensory input involves both sides of the brain working together and sharing information effectively. This bilateral integration and coordinated use of both hemispheres increases neural networking and maximises the potential for learning.

Midline Barriers

Midline barriers are imaginary lines or 'walls' that divide the body, from head to foot, into a right and left (vertical midline) and a top half from the bottom half at the waist (horizontal midline). They exist initially to encourage the young child to use both sides or halves of the body and develop muscle tone equally.

To move about freely and perform everyday tasks, the child needs to be able to spontaneously cross the middle of the body with both arms and legs, or bend at the waist. Tasks could include putting on shoes and tying of shoelaces, sweeping the floor, hitting a ball with a bat, reading and writing, playing ball games or picking something off the floor. A child with difficulties carrying out these tasks is exhibiting the tell-tale signs of a retained midline barrier.

Thus midline crossing and bilateral integration mutually reinforce each other. The more the child crosses the midline, the stronger the brain communication becomes, and the stronger the brain communication, the better the ability to cross the midline.

Lateral Dominance

Lateral dominance refers to the side of your body you use more frequently and adeptly, whether it is your eyes, ears, hands or feet. A lateral dominance, whether right or left is the optimal functional organisation of the brain, and they usually show up by the age of six or seven when the vertical midline barrier has been integrated.

Many people display a cross dominance pattern[12], where a person might be right-handed, but display a dominant left foot; or favour the right eye, but the left ear. Cross dominance is said to be a result of a brain disorganisation. While some people are able to cope with this, many display sensory processing and learning difficulties.

Spatial Orientation

Spatial orientation is like a sensory map in the child's brain, telling them where they are in relation to the three-dimensional space around them. Through sensory exploration, children learn spatial concepts like direction, distance and location.

The child discovers the joy of having a body with body parts that relate to each other; and that different tasks require different levels of effort. Their maturing vestibular system tells them if they are still or moving. Their visual perception sense tells them the size and shape of objects, helps build a neural network of images and retain a visual memory of objects. It also helps to develop peripheral vision which teaches them to plan and navigate their surroundings.

Developing good visual-spatial skills help the child differentiate shapes, such as the letters b, d, g, p, and q; and the numbers 69 and 96. They make reading, writing and spelling easier, and helps with understanding mathematical concepts, relating to shapes, symbols, dimensions, area, and ordering and arranging numbers.

---

[12] (Hannaford, 2011)

Physical Inactivity is a Global Problem

Research has shown that movement is essential for healthy development. It also shows that children who have been struggling with learning, social or emotional difficulties can overcome them by doing seemingly unrelated activities to reading and writing. They can do this by learning how to coordinate their bodies, integrating their sensory processing system, developing spatial awareness, midline and bilateral integration, body geography – essentially by moving!

Yet, more and more children are moving less. They are not getting the early motor stimulation required for optimal school success and the consequence of this is seen in the classroom with more and more children exhibiting learning difficulties.

Sedentary behaviour has become a growing concern. In 2020, the World Health Organisation declared physical inactivity as a global problem[13], and a leading cause of disease and disability. As a civilisation, we are relying more on machines for most of our manual work, we are driven everywhere, are hyper-connected with our noses buried in our phones and our eyes glued to the screen.

This has serious implications for the future of our children. It is time to bring healthy movement back into their lives.

---

[13] (WHO, 2020)

Chapter II

Sensory Integration Activities

The activities in this chapter are broadly categorised to serve as a guide, for we know that when one part of the body moves, many body systems are engaged and stimulated.

Beneficial movement activities are those that encourage the arms and legs to cross in front or behind the body, those that encourage the heads to be placed below the waist, those that encourage both sides of the body to work together, those that integrate the sensory system, and those that engage the hands, heart and head.

With careful supervision, most of these activities can be conducted as a whole class lesson. Specific one-on-one therapy activities are not the intention of this book, but the exercises may be used to supplement existing routines with the children in your care.

Warm Up Exercises

1. Magic Beans

Imagery: **The Magic Beans**[14]
One fine day, I went to a fair
I met an old lady selling her wares.
Magic spells and secret potions
Healing herbs and hand-made lotions.

I caught her eye
And she caught mine.
The lady smiled and bade me hither
And in my ear, she did whisper.

"Magic seeds I gift to thee
Care for them and you will see.
Joy and laughter it will bring
Sunshine, moonbeams, surprising things."

Thrilled at my discovery
I hurried home and did not tarry.
A bag of seeds for me to sow
Into the ground they must go.

Earth and sun, wind and rain
Weaving magic to swell the grain.
The roots take hold, the shoots unfold,
A wondrous sight I did behold.

---

[14] A poem I wrote for the children, based on the beans movement.

Magic beans of every kind
Growing tall and all aligned.
Waving about with great gusto
Greeting me with a big 'Hello'!

Beans and their Signature Moves

1. Jumping Beans

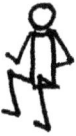

   - Jump up and down with both legs together, knees bent and tucked up high.

2. String Beans

   - Standing on tippy toes with hands reaching up high in the air.

3. Running Beans

   - Running on the spot as quickly as possible.

4. Broad Beans

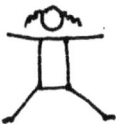

   - Jumping into a 5-pointed star, feet wide apart and arms horizontal.

5. French Beans

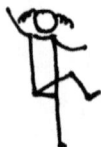

- Kicking feet across the midline, like dancing a can-can.

6. Hot Beans

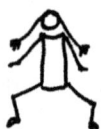

- Feet wide apart, step alternatively on each foot quickly as if on hot stones.

7. Jelly Beans

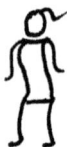

- Wiggle and jiggle as if like a jelly, shaking hands, wrists, legs, etc.

8. Climbing Bean

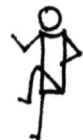

- With arms and legs, mimic the actions of climbing up a ladder.

9. Frozen Beans

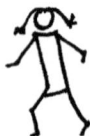

- Freeze on the spot.

10. Beans on Toast

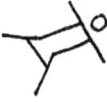

- Lying on the floor with feet wide apart, arms open out wide on either side.

11. Cross-Eyed Bean

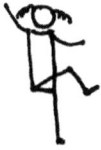

- Standing on tippy toes with feet crossed, one foot over the other, and arms crossed and raised overhead.

12. Three (or Four) Bean Salad

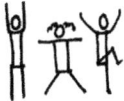

- Children divided into different groups of beans and by moving in character, gather into clusters of three or four different types of beans.

2. Puppet Carousel

Equipment: None

Skills: A great warm up exercise: Gross motor skills, attention, balance, coordination, quick reaction, crossing midline, bilateral integration archetypal movement patterns, vestibular stimulation.

Imagery: The children are little puppets on a carousel that goes round and round, sometimes forwards, sometimes back, sometimes staying on the spot, but all the while the little puppets are under the puppeteer's commands and they have to react quickly to the puppeteer's changing commands.

To Play: Children stand, spaced apart in a circle, facing inwards. Teacher gives command to turn right or left or face forward to move.

Commands: Use any combination of:

- Walking or running, forwards or backwards, sideways, stationary, turn around on the spot
- On tippy toes, heels, instep or outstep
- Skipping, galloping, trotting, crawling
- Hopping on one foot
- Hands or elbow to opposite knee / ankle
- Any of the bean greetings from exercise 1.

Option to play elimination – slowest person to react to changing command sits out and the last person standing is the winner; or after half the class is eliminated, the remaining group sits to rest while the eliminated group gets another chance to play carousel, but this time, without elimination.

Gross Motor Exercises

Equipment: Mostly none; bean bags and a basket;

Skills: Reflex integration, attention, balance, coordination, cross-ing midline, bilateral integration, vestibular stimulation, core muscle strength, gross motor.

1. Twinkling Toes

    • Lie on their back, with arms by their side. Tuck chin in towards chest, lift up head, and look at their twin-kling toes.

2. Worm in the Mud

    • Lie face down with arms by their sides, feet together, and chin tucked in towards chest. Engage core mus-cles, slowly extend (arch) the neck to lift the head and shoulders off the floor.

3. Airplane

    • Lie face down with arms bent at elbows, and legs straight. Tuck chin in and slowly lift head, chest, arms and legs off the floor.
    • Variation: arms are extended to the sides, legs straight but parted in a V shape.

4. Lizzy Lizard

    • Lie on their tummies, using arms and legs to help them move along the floor like a lizard.

5. Shooting Star

- Lie on backs, knees bent and feet flat on the floor. Press down on the feet and push off in the direction of the head like a shooting star (ensure safe space before starting).
- Reverse direction, by pulling with both feet together, moving towards the direction of the feet.

6. Pivoting on Tummy

- Lie on tummies with knees bent and legs in the air, use arms and core muscle strength to pivot around on the ground.

7. Walking on your Bottom

- Sit on their bottoms with legs straight out. Slowly shuffle with straight legs, moving forwards, backwards or to the sides.

8. Happy Baby

- Lie on their backs, bend and draw knees to chest, and hold on to the outside of feet or big toes. Gently massage backs by rocking sideways and in circles. Slowly release legs and rest. This is a great yoga pose that calms and quietens the mind.

9. Clapping with your Feet

- Lying on their backs, with feet in the air, clapping the soles of their feet together.
- Hand to feet clap – right hand to left foot and left hand to right foot.

10. Riding a Bicycle

- Lying on their backs, legs in the air, moving legs like riding a bicycle.

11. Dead Ants

- Lying on their backs with hands and legs in the air, shaking them like jelly.

12. Sand Angels

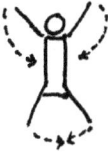

- Lying on their backs with arms by the side and legs together, sweep them out and in to form angel wings.

13. At the Zoo

- Children are animals and move around and make animal-like noises. Teacher calls out an animal and the children respond.
- Examples are snake slither, lizard crawl, seal drag, wombat walk, cat prowl, horse gallop, frog jump, bunny hop, penguin waddle, gorilla walk, elephant sway, bear walk, crab walk, bird flap, giraffe walk, deer prance, tiger prowl, flamingo hop, kangaroo bounce, inchworm crawl, cat stretch and cow pose.

Bilateral Integration, Eye-Hand Coordination, Midline Crossing and Concentration Exercises

Equipment: Bean bags, basket or hula hoops, two-metre-long elastics

Skills: Hand-eye coordination, crossing midline, bilateral integration, spatial awareness, gross and fine motor skills, attention, focus, concentration, rhythm and coordination, vestibular stimulation, motor planning.

1. Double Cross

    - Place bean bag on the head, cross arms at chest, and cross the feet.
    - Slowly squat down and stand up or sit down and stand up without dropping the bean bag or uncrossing hands and feet.
    - Repeat this five to ten times. For extra challenge, do it with eyes closed.

2. Toss, Clap and Catch

    - Hold bean bag in one hand, toss it, clap hands once before catching it.
    - Progress to two, then three claps etc. before catching.
    - Alternative: clap behind the back, or raise one knee and clap under the leg.
    - Instead of clapping, touch ears, shoulders, knees, or turn around once.
    - Catch bean bag with both hands, one hand, non-dominant hand or alternate hands.

3. Pat-a-Cake

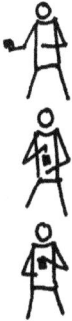

- Stand with arms bent, elbows by your side, palms facing upwards, and a bean bag in the left hand.
- Gently pass the bean bag back and forth across the body from one hand to the other, by turning the left hand over, whilst still holding on to the bean bag, and passing it on to the right hand. With bean bag now in the right hand, repeat the process by passing it to the left hand.
- In a circle or facing a partner: After passing the bean bag from the left hand to the right hand, the right hand now passes the beanbag to the outstretched left hand of the person to their right (or in front), while they receive a bean bag in their outstretched left hand from the person on their left (or in front).
- For suggestions of verses, see Appendix.

4. Round and Round

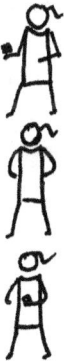

- Standing with arms bent, elbows by your side and palms facing upwards, and a bean bag in the right hand.
- Bring both hands behind the back and pass the bean bag from the right to the left hand. Bring both hands to the front and pass the bean bag with a little toss, from the left hand to the right. Repeat making rings around the waist.
- Move in rhythm to a song or verse, such as 'Mulberry Bush' (see Appendix).

5. Rainbow

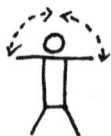

- Stand with arms open in the horizontal by the sides, palms facing upwards, and a bean bag in the right hand.
- Slowly bring both hands to meet above the head, passing the bean bag to the left hand. Bring arms to the horizontal with bean bag now in the left hand. Repeat, passing the bean bag the other way.
- Challenge: toss the bean bag from one hand to the other.

6. Under the Bridge

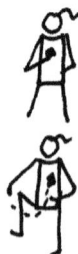

- Stand with arms by the sides, palms facing upwards and a bean bag in the left hand.
- Raise the left knee and toss the bean bag upwards under the left leg and catch it with the right hand as it falls. With bean bag now in the right hand, raise the right knee, toss it under the leg and catch with the left hand.
- Double bean bag: One bean bag in each hand, toss and catch with the same hand.
- Do it forwards and backwards, to counting, times tables, days of the week, letters of the alphabet, or in rhythm to verses[15].

7. Frogs on a Lily Pad

- Bean bags are little frogs jumping onto lily pads. Stand a short distance away, toss bean bags (underarm throw) into hula hoops. Try it with the non-dominant hand.

---

[15] See Appendix: Songs and Verses

- Upside down: with back to the hula hoop, bend the knees and fold forwards at the waist to look between the legs. Aim and toss bean bag into the basket.

8. Pinch your Nose and hold your Ears

    - Pinch your nose with one hand while the opposite hand crosses over the midline to hold your ear.
    - Switch hands, the hand holding the ear now pinches the nose and the hand pinching the nose now crosses the midline to hold the ear.

9. Pat your Head and Rub your Belly

    - Place one hand on your head and the other on your tummy.
    - Simultaneously pat your head gently and rub your belly.

10. Stepping Forwards and Backwards

    - This is a 1, 1; 1, 2, 1; 1, 2, 3, 2, 1; 1, 2, 3, 4, 3, 2, 1 pattern.
    - Stand with both feet together. Step right foot forwards and say aloud '1'. Transfer weight onto the back foot (*left* foot) to move backwards and say '1'.
    - To move forward, transfer weight onto the right foot and say '1', step the left foot forwards and say '2'. To move backwards, transfer weight onto the back foot (*right*) and count '1'.
    - To move forwards again, transfer weight onto the front foot (left) and count '1', step right foot forwards and say '2'; step left foot forwards and say '3'. To move backwards, transfer weight onto the back foot (*right* foot) and count '2', and step left foot backwards and say '1'.
    - Continue the sequence for as many counts as desired or feasible for your class.

- Added challenges:
  - clap hands in addition to the stepping and counting.
  - choose a number (e.g.'2') that is to be clapped, rather than spoken out loud: 1, clap, 3, 4, 3, clap, 1).
  - Step and recite days of the week, times tables or letters of the alphabet.

11. England, Ireland, Scotland, Wales (hand clap)

- Partners face each other, each placing their palms together, hands extended slightly to their right, fingertips pointing towards their partner, so that the back of their left hand touches the back of their partner's left hand.
- Partners tap hands in a to and fro manner, chanting the verse, accompanied by actions:

  England, Ireland, Scotland, Wales,
  Inside, Outside, Puppy Dog's Tails

- *England*: with hands together, partners tap the back of each other's left hands, continue through the motion so now their own hands are on the left side.
- *Ireland:* partners tap the back of each other's right hands, and return to starting position.
- *Scotland:* Partners tap the back of each other's left hands and stop.
- *Wales:* With the back of their left hands still touching, partners clap their own hands.
- *Inside:* keeping left hands in contact, partners bring their right hands up to clap each other's right hand.
- *Outside:* keeping left hands in contact, partners bring their right hands below their left hands to clap their partner's right hand.
- *Puppy Dog's:* Both partners cross clap their own knees (right hand to left knee, and left hand to right knee).
- *Tails:* Both partners to clap their own hands behind their own backs, like tails.
- Repeat the verse, going faster and faster.

12. England, Ireland, Scotland, Wales (elastics)

- You will require a continuous elastic band about 2 metres long[16] and two to three friends, taking turns. The objective is to jump nimbly without tripping.
- Stretch the elastic out between two players, around the ankles or calves.
- Jump in rhythm to the verse, accompanied by actions:
  England, Ireland, Scotland, Wales,
  Inside, Outside, Puppy Dog's Tails
- Begin by standing with both feet together on one side of the elastics lines.
- *England:* jump and land with right foot in and left foot to outside left of elastics.
- *Ireland:* Jump and land with left foot in and right foot to the outside right of elastics.
- *Scotland:* as for England.
- *Wales:* as for Ireland.
- *Inside:* Jump and land with both feet inside.
- *Outside:* Jump and land with both feet outside.
- *Puppy Dog's:* Jump and land with both feet inside.
- *Tails:* Jump and land with feet on elastics, right foot on right elastic and left foot on left side.
- Repeat going faster and faster.

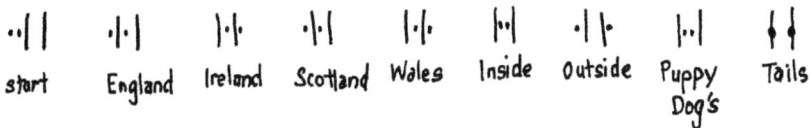

··| | ·|·|)·|·   ·|·| |·|· |·| ·| |· |··| ∤ ∤

start   England   Ireland   Scotland   Wales   Inside   Outside   Puppy   Tails
                                                                    Dog's

---

[16] As a child, I used to join rubber bands together to make the elastics.

13. London Bridge is Falling Down (elastics)

- Stretch a 2-metre-long elastic out between two players, around the ankles or calves.
- The third player jump in rhythm to the verse:
  London Bridge is falling down, falling down,
  falling down,
  London Bridge is falling down, my fair lady.
- Start with both feet on outside left of elastics.
  - *London:* jump and land with right foot in and left foot to outside left of elastics.
  - *Bridge:* jump and land with left foot in and right foot to the outside right of elastics.
  - *Falling:* jump and land with both feet in
  - *Down:* jump and land with both feet on elastics
  - *My:* jump and land with right foot in and left foot on outside left of elastics.
  - *Fair:* jump and land with left foot in and right foot on outside right of elastics.
  - *Lady:* jump and land with both feet on outside right of elastics in finishing position.

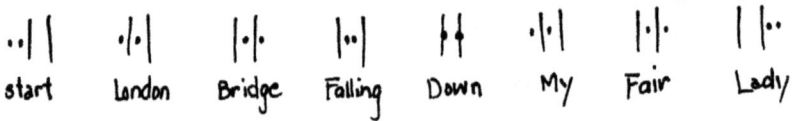

··│ │	·│·│	│·│·	│··│	┼┼	·│·│	│·│·	│ │··
start	London	Bridge	Falling	Down	My	Fair	Lady

14. Hickey Pickety (a straight line on the ground)

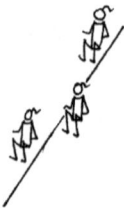

- Stand with both feet together, next to and parallel to a long straight line. Jump with both feet together to the opposite side, and back and forth repeatedly, travelling forward, up this line.

- For older children, jump moving backward to the start of the line, or criss-cross jumps (from about 10 years onwards when back space awareness is introduced).
- For suggested verse, see Appendix.

15. Rainstorm

- Like all families, Father Sky, Mother Earth, Sister Rain and Brother Wind sometimes talk gently to each other, taking turns and never interrupting or talking over each other. Sometimes they forget their manners and talk all at once, each talking over the other, each raising their voice. You know that is happening when you hear the pitter-patter of rain, the howling of the winds, the roaring of the waves and the thunderclaps in the air!
- Children stand in a circle, facing in.
- The teacher stimulates a rainstorm by performing a continuous action, which is simulated by the person on the right, and passed on to the next person on the right and so on, until everyone is doing the same motion.
- When the wave returns, the teacher changes the motion and passes it on. Keep the action going throughout the rainstorm, changing actions only when the person before you change their actions.
- Actions: begin and end with silence, going from soft and gentle to loud and energetic:
    - Silence, rub both hands together, snap fingers, pat thighs, stomp feet.
    - Then reverse the action: pat thighs, snap fingers, rub hands. Silence.

Vestibular Exercises

Equipment: Some require a partner, a balance beam, bean bags

Skills: Attention, balance, coordination, midline crossing, vestibular, core muscle strength, gross motor development

1. Roll, Roll, the Rolling Pin

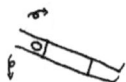

    - Lie on their backs with legs straight and arms extended above the head, like a log, and roll slowly to one side, and then reverse direction. Repeat several times.
    - Added challenge: roll with arms by their sides or arms crossed at chest.
    - Assists with transitioning between prone and supine positions. A word of caution: some children get dizzy, but with regular practice, it should decrease.

2. Catch a Falling Star (with partner and bean bag)

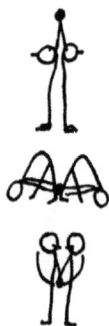

    - Stand back to back with a partner, with one partner holding a beanbag (the star).
    - Over and under pass: Pass the beanbag overhead to receiving partner, then both bend forwards, for receiving partner to return the bean bag, between the legs.
    - Side pass: Pass the beanbag by both twisting to the same side and then both twisting to the opposite side.

3. Row, Row, Row Your Boat (with partner)

- Sitting down facing a partner, and holding hands, the sailors rock to and fro.
- Great for vestibular stimulation, balance and control.

4. Bridge (with partner)

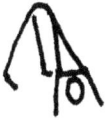

- Similar to the yoga pose 'Down Dog'.
- On hands and knees, curl toes under, straighten knees and lift up the hips, keeping head between arms. Now we have a human bridge. Option to have a partner who can crawl through.

5. Windmill

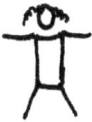

- Start with feet together and arms spread wide, slowly turn around 360° one way, several times, then repeat the other way.
- Make up a verse to go with it, such as:
    This is how the windmill goes
    round and round up and down
    This is how the windmill sounds
    Swish! Swish! Swish! Swish!

Fine Motor Exercises

It has been noted that in the animal kingdom, the more mobile and dexterous the extremities of an animal are, the more intelligent it is. It is in the hand that the human brain differentiates itself from other animals, and as they say, nimble fingers make nimble minds.

Equipment: Mostly none, paper and pencil

Skills: Fine motor dexterity, hand-eye coordination, rhythm and coordination.

1. A Walk in the Park

    • Fingers go for a stroll, by drumming across the floor or desk, arms stretching forwards and back.
    • Fingers explore the terrain (over their own faces, arms, legs, body).

2. Crab Crawl
    • Stretch your right arm across to the left side of your body, fingers spread out. Crab walk (thumb to pinkie, then extend pinkie) in an arc over to the right side of the body. Repeat with the left arm.

3. Finger Raisers

    • Here is the postman knocking at the door! Place palms of hand flat on the table. Lift thumb up and lower it, then repeat this with each finger in turn. See Appendix for suggested verse: Rat-a-tat.[17]
    • Helps with finger dexterity and increases the range of movement of the hands.

---

[17] See Appendix: Songs and Verses

4. Click go the Shears

   • With palms flat, spread fingers out and then close them, much like a sheep shearer clicking his shears as he snips the fleece off the sheep.

5. Sally Goes Round the Sun

   • Curl fingers in towards the palm, with the thumb resting over the tip of the pointer finger. Thumb makes circles over the tip of each finger (clockwise direction for right thumb and anticlockwise for left thumb).
   • Accompany with a song or verse[18].

6. Push and Pull

   • With arms horizontal at chest level: place both palms together, fingertips pointing up. Push as hard as possible against each other.
   • Pivot on the palms of the hand, so they come to rest, one palm over the other, at chest level. The fingertips of each hand curl, each hand griping the curled fingers of the other hand, and pull them in opposite directions.

7. Choo-Choo Train

   • Place a pencil between the palms of the hand, and roll it to and fro, making little "choo-choo" or "chug-chug" sounds.
   • Make up a story of a passenger train, starting and stopping.
   • The speed at which the train travels will vary when it slows down or stops to pick up more passengers, restarts and then travels at speed etc.

---

[18] See Appendix: Songs and Verses (Sally goes round the sun)

8. Incy Wincy Spider[19]

- Touch the tips of right-hand pinkie to the left thumb and the tips of the left-hand pinkie to the right thumb.
- Release right pinkie – left thumb connection, pivot on the right thumb – left pinkie, so the right pinkie and left thumb reconnect, moving in an upward motion. Repeat.
- Spider push ups: Place palms together, one hand is Incy, the other the mirror.
  - With fingertips and base of hand touching, slowly peel knuckles away to form a diamond shape. Open and close them or spread them wide, allow Incy to do his push-ups on a mirror.

9. Where is Thumbkin?

- A popular finger play[20] that helps children to isolate fingers and build awareness of their hand.
- Begin with right hand Thumbkin, followed by left hand Thumbkin, then each finger, sequentially on each side.

10. Fireflies a-Glowing

- Bending your elbows and holding your hand out in front, close both hands into a tight fist, then uncurl and spread fingers wide, like a flicker of firefly light. Repeat several times.
- For a silly ditty, perhaps consider this glow worm verse[21].

---

[19] Popular nursery rhyme. See Appendix: Songs and Verses (Incy Wincy Spider)
[20] See Appendix: Songs and Verses (Where is Thumbkin).
[21] See Appendix: Songs and Verses (Glow-worm)

11. Snow Ball Flick

- Take a piece of scrap paper, fold it in half and tear it. Repeat folding and tearing until you have eight pieces of paper. Scrunch them up and make little paper snowballs.
- Place a snowball on the palm of one hand. With the other hand, flick the snowball as far as you can, using each finger in turn. Swap hands and repeat the process.
- Make sure children collect all the little snowballs at the end of the lesson so it doesn't melt and leave a puddle on the floor.

12. Slowly, Slowly Creeps the Snail (with a rod)

- Curl one hand (the snail) around the base of the rod with the rod pointing up (garden rail).
- Working the fingers, slowly 'climb' to the top of the 'rail'. The hand does not move up, just the rod sliding downwards.
- When it reaches the top, slowly creep down the garden rail.
- Repeat with the other hand.
- Accompany this with a verse or song[22].

---

[22] See Appendix: Songs and Verses (Slowly, Slowly Creeps the Snail)

Feet and Toe Exercises

Each of our fingers is represented by its little section of the brain, and with frequent use, stimulates better coordination between the hand and brain. Our toes too, have a pathway to the brain, only they are not used to their full potential. Research with foot painters have shown that distinct areas of the brain 'lit up' when each toe of the dexterous foot is tapped, much like what happens when our fingers touch something.[23]

When we confine our feet to shoes, we restrict their freedom to explore. When children ask why I make them do toe exercises, I tell little stories about lighting up a Christmas tree or lighting candles to help find my way in the dark.

Equipment: Marbles, basket, a straight line, crayons or chalk

Skills: Fine motor dexterity, crossing midline, rhythm, balance and coordination,

1. Feet and Toe Yoga

   - Stand with feet together, slowly curl toes up and twinkle them, trying to splay the toes out to extend the gap between them. Release. Curl the toes under. Release.
   - Toe walk, one foot at a time, by curling the toes under, bring the heel towards the toes, then extend the toes and glide forwards. Toe walk backwards.
   - Up and down: Stand with feet together, slowly raise the heels, pressing toes into the ground, then slowly lower the heels.
   - Forwards and backwards: Slowly tilt backwards pressing heels into the ground without raising the toes off the floor. Slowly shift weight forwards to press the toes into the ground, without raising the heels off the floor.

---

[23] (Cohut, 2109)

2. Hungry Feet

   • Place marbles on a carpeted surface. Children use their feet to pick up marbles and place them into a container across their midline to the right or left, or into a small container a short distance away.
   • How hungry are their toes? How many marbles can their feet pick up at any one go? Are both feet hungry?

3. Wiggle Marbles with Toes

   • Sit on the floor. With fingers, place a marble in the web space between the big and second toe, and wriggle toes to dislodge the marble.
   • Next, place it between the second and third toe, and wriggle the marble out. Repeat for the other toes.
   • Do this with both feet individually or simultaneously.

4. Marble Bowling

   • This is a 'feet' only game.
   • Lay a row of marbles of different sizes on a carpet, close together but not touching.
   • Stand a few paces away, and with your feet, pick up a 'bowling' marble and try to 'bowl' the line of marbles out, one at a time.
   • Make a game out of it and set your own rules.

5. Drawing with Toes (with crayons or chalk)

   • Tape a large sheet of paper on the floor. Place a block or stick crayon (or colour pencil) between the big and second toes and get creative. Try it with the other feet. Try it simultaneously, sitting on a chair, with two pieces of paper, one for each foot.

Chapter 3

Why Play Games?

The importance of children's play was highlighted in a 1560s painting, 'Children's Games'[24] by Flemish Renaissance artist, Pieter Bruegel. It depicts about 200 children in a town square playing over 80 different games, some of which are easily recognisable: tug of war on horsebacks, hobby horses, blind man's bluff, run the gauntlet, marbles, leap frog, top spinning, broom balancing, barrel riding, playing with dolls, carrying an angel (hand seat).

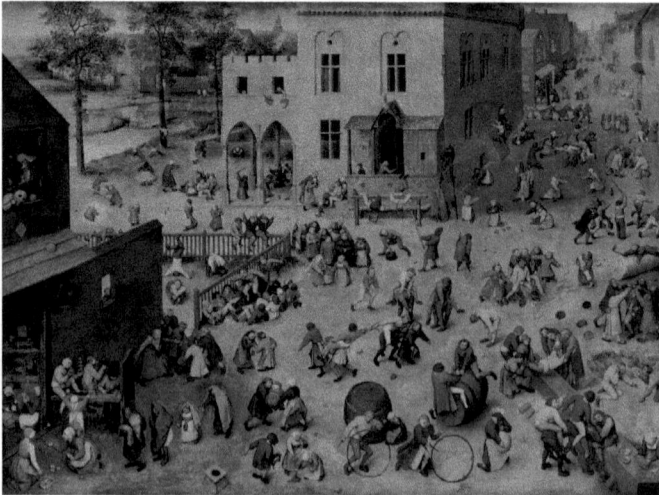

Children's Games by Pieter Bruegel the Elder. 1560. Oil on panel. 118 cm × 161 cm). Reproduced here with permission from KHM-Museumsverband.

---

[24] (Bruegel, 1564) held and exhibited at the Kunsthistorisches Museum in Vienna.

The opportunity to play is the opportunity to work, and in fact, play is the child's work. Recent studies[25] have shown that play is crucial to enriching the child's physical, social, intellectual and emotional development.

---

[25] (Dr White, 2012), (Playground Professional, 2015) (Johnson, 1907 reprinted 2015)

Play as an Educational Tool

As an educational tool, playing games is simple, yet so profound. Games enliven the imaginative life of the child. Through free play and games, children find their own learning situations, and they consider different outcomes to situations they encounter.

Games develop alertness and resourcefulness. Children learn to sense the danger of being tagged or when the ball is coming their way. They feel the touch on their shoulder, they hear their name being called and they learn to dodge with agility.

Games teach moral and social values. Children learn to communicate and relate socially; to take turns, value teamwork and cooperation; to not monopolise opportunities and to be selfless in sacrificing oneself for the sake of the team. They learn honesty by owning up to being tagged, and that games are not about winning at all cost.

Games foster critical thinking and problem solving. Children are able to exercise and consolidate their ability to understand, think, appreciate, and develop concentration. They learn to find ways to accomplish their goal.

Games build confidence and self-esteem. When skills and challenges are achievable and age appropriate, children gain the confidence they need for future challenges. They practice ball handling skills in a game of tag or chase, rather than focusing on the physical 'skill' activity itself, thus reducing self-consciousness or awkwardness.

Games train the development of willpower and endurance. Children who tumble when being chased learn to get up, brush off their fall and try again. They learn to take safe 'risks' and give 'dares' in capturing an opponent or in rescuing team member.

Games grow resilience. Children learn to regulate their own needs and those of others. When one is tagged and has to sit out, by doing so, one allows the game to go on so others can play. They learn to take defeat with grace, bear the pangs of being 'caught' or of not being 'it'.

Games grow character. They learn to exercise self-control and restraint in their interactions with others. They learn to be respectful of rules of engagement, to not act impulsively and emotionally and to be accountable for their actions.

Research [26] has shown that 'good players', those with the ability to play with others, show more empathy and compassion, have increased social skills, and are better able to see things from another's perspective.

Games bring health to the body and joy to the spirit, and are the heart of education for the growing child!

---

[26] (Bancroft, 1909)

The Healing Forces of Imagination

Imagination may seem like a frivolous activity on the outside, but when children use their imagination in play, they are developing crucial cognitive and social skills.

When we imagine, we activate the amygdala (the part of the brain associated with emotions) and the cortex (where logical processes take place). The best learning takes place when we engage the whole body: muscles, thoughts, emotions and imagination[27]. Think of imagination as a muscle. If we do not exercise it, it will not flourish!

Between the ages of seven to fourteen, children live in a world of vivid imagination. They think poetically, in imagery, and are capable of inspired insights. Theirs is a 'feeling' kind of thinking, which progresses to more abstract and analytical thinking.

Storytelling engages children's imagination and strengthens their inner picturing capabilities. Like the wisdom of fairy tales, stories can have transformative, healing and educative powers[28]. They stimulate feelings and allow children to process and come to terms with the dilemmas of inner life.

Games become vivid and alive when children imagine themselves to be pirates sailing the sea, knights slaying dragons or sheep being chased by wolves. Here, they learn to confront the evil, the bully or the greedy, and overcome them. If we foster and nurture this capacity, and allow children the time, space and opportunity to live into the pictures and experiences presented to them, they can carry this strong power of imagination into their adult life.

Movement for the sake of movement is soulless, but when imbued with joy and imagination, it is healing for body, soul and spirit.

---

[27]   (Nielsen, December 6, 2010)

[28]   (Kornberger, 2013)

Developmental Approach to Education

Children unfold in a way that is quite universal, judging from their physical characteristics, growth, play, imagination, imitation, emotions, drawings, ideals, purposes, feats, ambitions, interests, and relationship to the space around them. Each phase has significance and value in relation to education[29].

This unfolding follows the path of the evolution of consciousness in humanity, recapitulating in a general way the earliest forms of consciousness, and advancing to the modern. A helpful way for us as parents and teachers, is perhaps to reflect on what the child standing before us, year to year, might ask, "Who am I as a learner?" and "What is my place in this world right now?"

Teaching is a balance between knowing what supports the general development of the child at a particular age and knowing what the child needs at that moment. A movement curriculum needs to be informed by this understanding.

The teacher of movement and games, when working creatively and imaginatively, may reach the children by stimulating their imagination. If we are able to return to childhood with them, and teach with delight, joy and imagination, then we will have reached them on a soul level.

Recognising that children have an unfolding consciousness, a growing awareness of, and ability to relate to the world around them means that the teacher has to find a way to relate to children at each year level. How can the teacher do it?

---

[29] (Johnson, 1907 reprinted 2015)

The Sheaths of Authority

The sheath of authority is concerned with "who am I as a teacher?" and "how do I establish my authority to maintain discipline, yet meet the incarnating needs and intellectual development of the children?"

Children need a teacher who knows what they need[30]. Teachers need to set appropriate boundaries for children's age and development, give clear directions, maintain consistency and strive for fairness, so that children are free to fully engage in class activities. There will be no anxiety over what behaviours are deemed appropriate or inappropriate, and children will be able to flourish.

In the primary school years, children respond best to a 'loving authority' cultivated by the teacher, allowing them to learn in a natural and developmentally beneficial way[31]. There is no readymade discipline solution, nor should there be a 'one size fits all' approach. It is the teacher's responsibility to intuit what is needed for the situation and class.

Dan Freeman[32] suggests assuming a 'sheath of authority', which is like an invisible cloak or sheath that the teacher 'wears', or an 'aura' that the teacher personifies, when dealing with the children. This authority should be evident to the children and it changes or develops with the children's development. This is described in more detail in games for each year level.

---

[30] Titus Witsenburg (personal communication)

[31] (Hartman, 2013)

[32] Dan Freeman, from his lectures and personal communication.

Games Origins and Categories

Both Johnson[33] and Bancroft[34], in their extensive research, have concluded that very few games are of modern invention, and that many can be traced back to antiquity, to some forms of religious or initiation ceremonies. Many of these have been analysed, adapted and graded for educational purposes, for example Bancroft (1909). They in turn have been passed down, further adapted, and varied, with the addition of what Bancroft (1909) calls 'local colour'. For example, 'Cat and Mouse' appears in some cultures as 'Wolf and Lamb', and I have adapted some games to include animals native to Australia, such a 'Dingo and Possum' instead of 'Fox and Rabbit".

The games in this book cover some common types, including

- fundamental movement skills (e.g. basic running, skipping, gross motor movement)
- basic chasing and fleeing (tag)
- invasion (invading another team's space or play area)
- target (e.g. the sending of an object towards a target)

Basic Tag Games

Tag games involve chasing and fleeing, and they are universally popular, especially with younger children. There are many variants, but they all follow some basic principles:

- One or more persons is designated 'It'.
- 'It' chases and tries to 'tag' others, who try to flee from 'It'.
- A 'tag' is a touch with the hand, or a hit with a ball or other object specified. It is NOT a forceful, spiteful or mean contact in any way. For older children, some rough play may be part of the game, but never in a mean way.

---

[33] (Johnson, 1907 reprinted 2015)
[34] (Bancroft, 1909)

- 'Tagged' player may become 'It' / be eliminated / sit out for a specified time / be given an alternate role / do a penalty / join Tagger in a chain tag.
- A chain tag is a build-up – when 'It' tags someone, they join hands, to become 'It'. As more people are tagged, they are added to 'It' and the chain grows. A variation is for a chain of four to split into two.
- Tag games can also be played in teams.
- I like giving 'It' an identity, a soul, a story that enlivens children's play. Instead of saying 'You are 'It', I choose to tell them a story and then say, for example, "Now, you are the Shark!"

Basic Invasion Games

These are usually team games, requiring teams to invade each other's play area or space, in order to score points (or achieve a goal), while keeping the opposing team's score to a minimum. Sports like soccer, hockey, rugby and basketball utilise the elements of invasion tactics.

The skills and strategies required in invasion games include teamwork and cooperation, defending team space or objects, attacking the opponents' space and retrieving objects, anticipation, ball handling skills, dodging, change of direction, speed and agility, spatial awareness and problem solving. These skills are transferrable to everyday life.

Invasion games are very popular with children from the upper primary levels. They are eager and ready to transition to team sports and relish the opportunity to test their developing physical, social and cognitive abilities.

How to Create Your Own Games?

Once you understand children's developing needs, it is not difficult to create your own game. Consider some of the game elements below. Then all you need is a handful of inspiration, a spoonful of enthusiasm, a dash of creativity, a pinch of intuition, a sprinkling of humour, a smidgen of drama, and a dollop of fun. Try it!

- formation (e.g. circle, line or opposing groups)
- modes of contest (is it 1 vs 1; 1 vs group, group vs group)
- type of contest (e.g. is it a test of strength, skill, speed, agility balance, or a combination)
- objective (e.g. to be the first or last; to beat the clock; to get across safely; to rescue, capture or defend; to decimate; to keep a ball aloft; to collect the most; to get rid of the most)
- methods of capture (e.g. touch tag, ball tag, wrestle)
- concealment and detection (e.g. hide, seek, disguise)
- challenges (e.g. time, distance, location, territory, goal, roles, physical, danger)
- types of props (e.g. ball, hula hoops, bean bags, mats, plank)
- type of movement (e.g. run, jump, hop, skip, kick, throw, pull, drag, balance, aim, clap in rhythm, wrestle, dodge)
- elimination and redemption (can they re-join the game?)
- penalty (e.g. do sit ups, star jumps, toss a beanbag)
- suspense (e.g. when will it be revealed, how long to wait, who will reveal, how will it be revealed?)
- handicaps (e.g. throwing with non-dominant hand, pegged legged, blindfolded, link hands with partner)

For example, I created the game 'Three Billy Goats Gruff' to address core muscle tone issues for a class of 8-year-olds. Then incorporate imagery, suspense, a protagonist, a hero, a rescue effort, and a catchy title. Have fun creating your own games. Very often the children will help with their own variations.

Managing Games with Children

The gym or outdoor play area is an extension of the teacher's classroom, and many factors can impact a lesson's outcome. All teachers have their own unique methods for teaching, discipline and management of games, and the suggestions in this section, is borne out of experience, and may be helpful to the novice or beginning teacher or games facilitator.

Meeting the Children

Meet the children on common ground by engaging in the games with them. Nothing gains the respect and affection of a child more than a grown up person showing an interest in, and participating in their games. The children will open their hearts to them. This in turn enhances the teacher-pupil relationship, giving the teacher further insight into the nature of the child.

When choosing a game, look at each situation and what the children need at that time. Repeating a game can be more valuable than choosing a new game every time.

Establishing Boundaries

A physical boundary or perimeter helps ensure a safe, obstacle and hopefully, distraction free, place to play. Children can see the space and feel held.

Social and interactional boundaries ensure everyone understands what is acceptable behaviour and what is not, for example a 'tag' is gentle but firm, and not forceful and mean.

Teacher's expectation is another boundary. Gather the children with a command that works for you (e.g. "Huddle up") and be consistent with its use. Give them a time limit (e.g. 5 seconds) to gather and do what is expected when you give the command (e.g. sit, look, listen).

Negotiating Rules

Game rules are like a temporary social contract, and they may change with circumstance, or with age and maturity, for example the game 'Cat and Mouse' has many versions and children learn to abide by the rules of the version that they are playing.

There are also consequences attached to those rules, for example, stepping out of boundary during a tag is the same as being tagged.

Some rules are negotiable, for example, whether tagging another child's hair is considered a tag; whether tagging is below the shoulder, or waist or knee; or whether steps taken towards 'Mr Wolf' are running steps or walking steps, as long as they are clear and everyone abides by them. Learning to negotiate is an important part of the games process and helps develop social skills.

The adult's role is that of an arbitrator (if negotiations between children get stuck), an enforcer (of whatever the current rules are) and a motivator (to seed ideas or provide impulse if children are slow to motivate)[35].

Presenting the Game

Most children benefit from a full explanation, followed by a walk through or demonstration of the game. Add a story or image and the game comes alive. Seeing a game actively demonstrated allows children to learn though imitation. It also strengthens their will by seeing what needs to be done and setting out to achieve it.

Avoid teaching and playing a game at the same time, unless it is a large and disorderly group, and the only way to deal with it is to gain their interest and attention, then halt for further explanation.

When the game involves a ball, I might have a 'talking ball' where the person with the ball may do the talking or ask a question. This teaches the children to listen respectfully and be listened to respectfully in return.

---

[35] Freeman (training notes)

Make the game challenging but achievable. Always introduce the most basic, achievable version first before adding progressively more complicated versions.

Always have a safe zone, for example, a 'home', 'burrow' or 'den', and that children know the consequences of being out of the safe zone (i.e. falling into shark infested waters is the same as being tagged).

Elimination from a game can be painful, and inclusive versions of games give participants a way back in, or an alternate role. I use an in/out queue, for example, when they are tagged by the wolf, they go into the wolf's lunch box, and re-join the game when the fifth child is placed in the lunch box, pushing the first child out.

Games should have a clear beginning and an end that is understood by all. For example, when the Cat catches the Mouse, they swap roles; or the team that catch all the players of another team is the winner. For games without a clear ending, like when tagged children sit out and re-join the game after a time, ensure that children understand how you will call an end to the game.

Involve children in setting up and packing away the equipment. This gives them ownership of the game and develops social responsibility. However, there are times when the setting up sets the scene for the game, and the younger classes love to come into a gym where the obstacles are set up and a story waiting for them.

Emphasise self-development, participation, fair play and cooperation. Acknowledge when moral and social qualities are observed. Close the session by reviewing what worked and what didn't, and how it could be better, safer or fairer.

Practice inclusivity. An injured child may still be part of the game, for example, being the cherry on top of the cake, in 'Cut the Cake', or they are the Witch Doctor who is able to cure any illness, or a rock behind which the fishes hide from the shark.

Most importantly, enjoy and have lots of fun. Use humour as a tool to engage interest, reduce tension or even to resolve conflicts.

How to choose 'It'

There will always be children clamouring to be 'It', and those who need a little encouragement. I have used the following ways successfully:

- Rewarding good behaviour (this is broad enough to encompass helpfulness, sportsmanship, respect, courtesy, honesty, etc.).
- Welcoming a new child to the class.
- Celebrating a child's birthday.
- Encouraging a child, but giving them the option to say no. It may help to have a silent and unobtrusive gesture (e.g. arms clasped over their chest) for a child to indicate that they are not ready to be chosen as a protagonist.
- Choosing a child most suited to start a particular game (e.g. a quick runner or one who can quickly grasp the situation).

How to choose teams

Whichever methods you choose, do not be predictable! The older children are quick to read you and will always try to find ways to out-think you.

- Make a circle or a line and every alternate person stepping forward. This creates two circles or groups.
- Number them off '1', '2', '1', '2' etc., and all the '1's form a team and all the '2's form the other team. (or number them off for as many teams as required).
- Children pair up with the person next to them and play a game of 'Paper, Scissors, Rock'. The winners form a team and the rest form the other team.
- Heads or Tails: Children display Head (palms down) or Tail (palm up). Those who display Heads form one team and those with Tails form the other team. Adjust with a second game or clause to balance the numbers in the groups.

- For three groups, all play Paper, Scissors, Rock, and group them according to what they display. Again, you might need to tweak or adjust to even the numbers in the group.
- Teacher 'randomly' selects the groups. I mentally pair up two students of equal ability, and select one for each group, keeping the teams as balanced as possible in regards to height, build and compatibility, etc.
- Random picks – those whose birthdates fall on an even number, those whose birth month is an even number, those wearing a certain colour shirt, those who have a pet dog, etc. Add a second or third clause if needed to get an even number of players in each team.
- Those seated by rows or side of the room.

How NOT to choose teams / pick a partner

- Captain's Pick: I avoid picking team captains and allowing them to pick their team members. This usually results in the strongest or fastest players being picked first leaving the other students feeling very deflated.
- Boys vs Girls: I avoid this for the younger groups, but there comes a time from Year 5 when the students request for this. It works for some groups, and not for others. Use your discretion.
- 'Choose a partner': For some children, and even adults, this method may induce fear, anxiety and embarrassment. They may start to question: What if they say no? What if they do not like me? What if I am left out? Some children are the 'preferred' candidates for partners and tensions may arise when two or more children wish for the same partners. This method can work if the group is sufficiently socially mature, are comfortable with each other, or if the activity requires constant changing of partners, so use your discretion.

When to Introduce Sports?

Games allow one to create, recreate and adapt, and the objective is to be inclusive and have fun. Sports, on the other hand, are formalised games with firm rules and strategies that usually involve competition, and the objective is to win. They pit one against another, or one team against another. Skills are defined and specific, and can be trained with discipline and structure.

When is your child ready for organised competitive sports? This question is not new and is much debated.

For some, it is 'the sooner the better' in the hope that if their child learns and develops the basic skills of the chosen sport early, they have a better chance of playing at a high level later on. Some parents go as far as engaging one on one coaching to provide extended training sessions for their children; advice on eating right and to engage in competition at the highest level, in the hopes of a glorious athletic career[36].

Many sports competition and training begin as early as six years of age[37]. Proponents suggest that children from 8 years old are ready for competitive sports and little leagues, and are in a better positon to 'handle the stresses of winning, losing, and being measured and scored on their performance'.[38]

As adults and educators, it is our responsibility to ask: Are our children mini adults? Are they developmentally ready, physically, psychologically, emotionally and socially? Have they developed sufficient perceptual-motor skills? Are they ready for the trauma of defeat or sitting on the sidelines? Are they ready for the recurrent practice, drills and the acquisition of specific skills and concepts?

There are adverse effects to early specialization of one sport, such as missing out on development in other more generalised skills, mental well-being

---

[36] (Ballard, 2020)

[37] (Maffulli, 2000)

[38] (Holecko, 2020)

(increase anxiety and stress, isolation, less family time), insufficient sleep, burnout and injuries.[39]

When considering competitive sports for your child, I urge parents to ask themselves: "Is it about me or about my child? Am I imposing my adult values into my child's play? Am I competing against other adults through my child?"

Every child is different, and some are naturally gifted, intrinsically endowed and motivated to be able to withstand the rigours of intense training. There are children, who for a variety of reasons, respond to the need to play certain sports, and that is their calling.

But for most children, development should not be rushed, but enhanced with age appropriate activities and experiences. Competitive sport should not begin before adolescence[40], at about twelve years of age. That is when they are ready for law, order and structure. Drawing a parallel between the developing consciousness of the human being and the evolution of society and culture throughout history, that epoch is that of the Roman Empire, a class six curriculum in the Steiner Schools.

What is age appropriate experience? Begin with free play, and imaginative play, indoors and out; to games with flexible rules with no winners or losers, then to informal teams with flexible rules that emphasise fun and that acts as a transition to organised team sports.

In a sport mad culture, like Australia, it is inevitable that many children will be involved in sport much earlier than twelve years old. Adults carers should bear in mind that children may not fully understand the strategies, but will do their best to please the coach, their parents or peers. Enjoyment and skill development must always have priority over winning[41].

---

[39]   (Dr Geier, 2020)

[40]   (McMillan, 2019) (Kischnick, 1979), Freeman (lecture notes) (Brooking-Payne, 1998)

[41]   Freeman (lecture notes)

Chapter 4

Games by Year Level

Children's capacity to deal with physical, social, emotional, and intellectual challenges unfold with age and experience. A movement curriculum needs to be informed by this understanding, and nothing should be brought in before they are ready to process them

The games in this chapter are listed by age and school year level. Each year level begins with an overview of the developmental picture of the child at that age, the movement emphasis and the teacher's sheath of authority. They are given as guides, not dogma, can be played from that age or year level onwards, even into adulthood. Please choose the games that resonate with you and the children and modify or adjust as required.

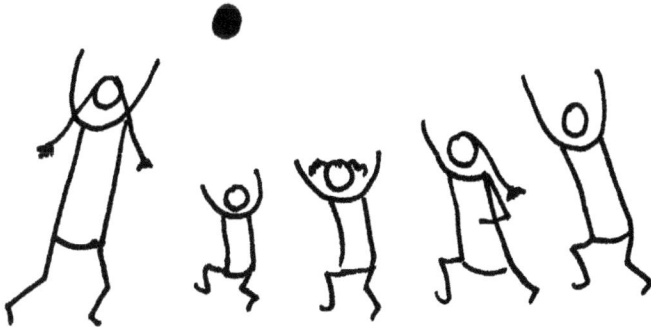

Year One: (Ages 6 to 7)

Developmental Picture of the Seven-Year-Old:

Dreamy

The child is still a little dreamy, and lives in a world filled with colour, fantasy and imagination. They respond to learning through pictorial and rhythmic activities, and through imitation. Many things do not touch the child because they cannot yet be reached intellectually and emotionally. Their ability to focus is developing.

The child needs security and support for their emerging independence; to experience themselves as a whole, yet connected to their environment, and the ability to relate to what they experience.

Images help nurture this sense of wholeness and allows the child to internalise lived experiences, which in turn help with recall and then the ability to transform perceptions into concepts.

Movement Emphasis for Year 1

- Focus is to develop fine and gross motor ability, spatial awareness and social skills.
- Games should be played within an imaginative context, contain an archetypal character or a song/rhyme and movement.
- Children at this age do not like to be confronted by a group, so do not single them out in a one against the group scenario. The Teacher should be the protagonist, otherwise, have two or more take on the role (e.g. 2 : All or group vs group). Find a way for children to silently indicate to you if they are not ready to be a protagonist (e.g. by clasping their hands over their chest).
- Circle formation is ideal.

The Teacher's Sheath of Authority:

Fairy King or Queen

The six to seven-year-old is still in a dreamy realm, and the teacher's role is to form a cohesive group, with respect for their abilities and authority. The teacher aims to provide a safe space for the children to grow and does so by captivating them with imagination and nourishing them with moral goodness appropriate for this age. And what does this authority look like? Why, that of the Fairy King or Queen[42]! The archetypal image of someone who works magic to cultivate the group soul.

Fairies are born of imagination and are in every folk lore. They are pure of spirit, helpful and benevolent and are known to watch over the land. The Fairy King or Queen rules over his magical classroom with a leadership that is calm, soothing, graceful, yet sparkly and creative and attentive to the children's needs. All cannot help but be captivated by his or her authority, and follow instructions happily and cheerfully.

---

[42] Dan Freeman (personal communication)

1. Heads Down Thumbs Up

Equipment: None

Skills: Tactile, sensory integration, eye-hand coordination

Imagery: Tiny Tom Thumb is no larger than one's thumb! His play mates are little Elfin fairies who are no larger than he is, and they love to play a guessing game with his human friends. Can you guess which Elfin fairy has chosen to play with you today?

To play:
- Children are seated at their desks, or around a circle. Choose three to five children as Elfin fairies, who stand in front of the class.
- Teacher calls *'Heads down, thumbs up!'*, and seated children rest their heads on their desk, their eyes closed and thumbs sticking up.
- Elfin fairies walk around quietly, each choosing someone whose thumb they gently push down, then return to the front of the room.
- Teacher calls 'Heads up, thumbs down'. Children chosen by the Elfin fairies guess who chose them.
- The player who guesses correctly swaps places with the Elfin fairy for the next round. Elfin fairies not caught out may go for the next round.

Variations:
- 'Heads up, stand up' gets everyone standing up.
- Limit each Elfin fairy to a maximum of two rounds each turn.

2. Duck, Duck, Goose (Grey Duck)

Equipment: None

Skills: Gross motor, awareness, attention, quick reaction

Imagery: Once upon a time, there was a little duckling, who was teased about being ugly because she was grey, and not the pretty yellow like all the other ducklings in the pond. Some even called her 'goose!'. But little grey duck held her head high. When they chased her, she would chase them back to show that she was just as special. As the ducklings grew older, it turned out that little grey duckling was really a cygnet, who is now transformed into a beautiful and graceful swan.

To play:
- All children sit in a circle, facing inward, except one child (the tagger) who walks around the outside of the circle.
- The tagger touches each child lightly on the head, each time saying "Duck". Nothing happens when they say "Duck" but when they say "Goose", the chase is on. The Goose chases the tagger who tries to run around the circle to take the seat vacated by the Goose.
- If the tagger successfully returns to the spot, the Goose becomes the new tagger. If the tagger gets caught, the Goose remains the tagger and tries again. If the tagger does not succeed a second time, assign a new tagger.

3. I wrote a Letter

Equipment: A handkerchief or small object

Skills: Gross motor, attention, quick reaction

Imagery: Little Lucy wrote a letter to her grandma. She was on her way to the post office when she unknowingly dropped it. You can imagine her distress when she found out! So Little Lucy skips around town, asking if anyone has found the letter.

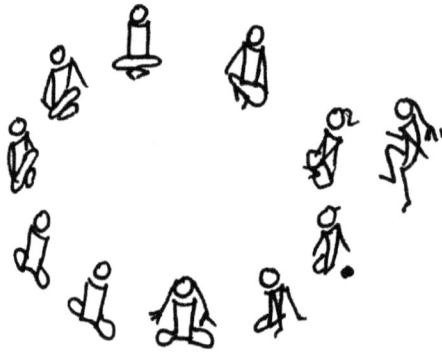

To play:
- Children sit crossed legged in a circle facing inwards. One child is Little Lucy, who stands on the outside of the circle, with a letter in her hands (a handkerchief). She skips around singing (to the tune of Yankee Doodle):
  "I wrote a letter to my grandma. On the way I dropped it. Someone must have picked it up and put it in his pocket. Please, please, drop it x3"
- Little Lucy drops the handkerchief behind someone in the circle and skips away while being chased by the person now with the hanky. The first person back to the vacated spot is safe, and the other becomes Little Lucy for the next round.
- The game ends at the Teacher's discretion.

4. Thread the Needle

Equipment: None

Skills: Spatial orientation, teamwork

Imagery: Gargantua, the good natured giant has a hole in his shirt. The good fairies have found a giant needle and some rainbow coloured thread to help him mend his shirt. But first they need to thread the needle.

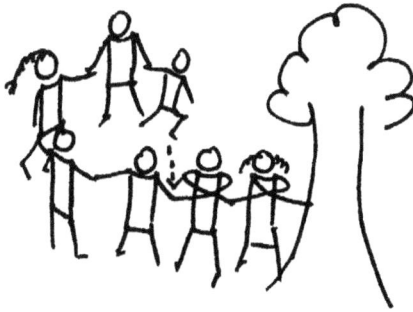

To play:
- Children are the thread and they stand in a long line, holding hands.
- The first child stands next to a tree or a wall, and puts their free hand up against it, making an arch (the eye of the needle).
- The end child runs through this arch, pulling the rest of the children along, except for the first child, who without letting go of the next child's hand or contact with the tree, turns 180° so that their arms are crossed over their chest.
- Repeat the process through the arch formed by the first and second child. This time, the second child turns 180° and stands next to the first child with their arms crossed over their chest.

- Continue until all players are standing the other way round with arms crossed over.
- To test the strength of their stitching, the first and last child link hands, facing inwards, and the circle moves in a clockwise direction. At a signal from the Teacher, they pull backwards to see if the chain breaks.

Variations:
- The eye of needle can also be in the middle, with the arch formed by the middle two children, with both ends running through at the same time.

5. Red Light, Green Light

Equipment: None

Skills: Gross motor, spatial awareness, listening, attention

Imagery: Once upon a time, there were three good friends, Right Light, Green Light and Yellow Light. Red Light is short and stern, Green Light is happy and cheerful and Yellow Light is slow and careful. Despite the difference in their personality, the three friends got along very well together, making life easy for everyone on the road.

To play:
- All the children are cars, standing in a line at one end of the play area. The teacher is the Traffic Lights, standing at the opposite end of the play area, just beyond the finishing line.
- Before beginning, the teacher clarifies the rules: the children move forwards on Green Light, stop on Red light and slow down on Yellow Light.
- The teacher gives the commands and the children respond. The objective is for all (or most) to cross the finish line before the game begins anew.
- Those who do not slow down or stop as required, have to return to the start line.
- The teacher may specify how the children move on Green Light (e.g. walk, run, skip, hop, gallop; or Yellow Light (e.g. walk heel to toe)

6. Hot Potato Toss

Equipment: One bean bag or soft foam ball

Skills: Throwing and catching skills, spatial awareness

Imagery: Hot baked potatoes are really yummy, but fresh out of the oven, they are very, very hot and can burn your hands. Sometimes, greedy children forget to wait for them to cool and "Ouch!" they get a potato burn, and have to sit out for first aid. So if a hot potato comes your way, toss it away!

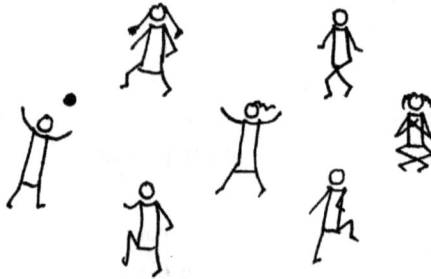

To play:
- Children stand in a random manner around the play area. One child begins by tossing a bean bag to another child who has to catch it.
- A child who throws the bean bag poorly or who misses a catch has to perform a penalty (sit out for the count of 10) before re-joining the game.

Variations:
- Vary the penalty – e.g. cross arms and legs and sit down and stand up again for ten times, without uncrossing limbs.
- Increase the level of difficulty when children are more confident of this game: all standing on one leg; clap once before a catch; catch with one hand; catch with non-dominant hand/ times table.

7. Crows and Cranes[43]

Equipment: None

Skills: Attention, memory, gross motor, agility

Imagery: Many years ago, Mr. Crow and Mr. Crane were friends, but one day, they had a fight! Mr. Crane had just caught a fish in the river when hungry Mr. Crow came by. Impatient, Mr. Crow refused to wait till it was cooked, and tried to steal some fish. Mr. Crane caught the fish in time and hit Mr. Crow in the eye with it so hard that he fell onto the coals. When he got up, he was black as crust, with a white patch over his eye.

Upset, Mr Crow was determined to get his back on Mr Crane. He took the fish bone and in the night, snuck up on a sleeping Mr Crane and placed the fish bone in his throat. When Mr Crane woke up the next morning, he started to complain, but alas, instead of his sweet voice, all that he could cry was "Gah-rah! Gah-rah!"

And that is how it came to be that Crows are black and Cranes cry "Gah-rah! Gah-rah!". To this day, Crows and Cranes have never forgiven each other and continue to play tricks on each other.

---

[43] A popular game whose origins I am unable to discover. This story is based on an Aboriginal folk tale, from (Dascy, 1930)

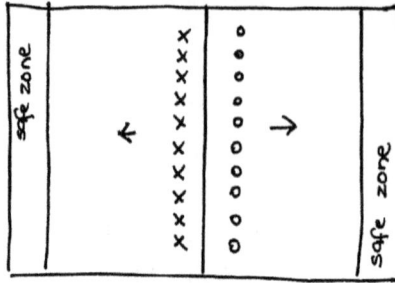

To play:
- Two equal groups, the Crows and the Cranes, stand back to back along a centre line (the river), each group on one side of the line. At either end of the play area is each group's safe zone.
- Teacher calls either "Crrrrrrows!" or "Crrrrrranes!".
- Whoever is called has to cross the river to chase the other group and tries to tag them before they reach their safe zone. Tagged players join their tagger's team for the next chase.
- The game ends when everyone is on one team.

Variations:
- Call "Crrrrrab" and everyone has to stay still. Anyone that moves has to join the opposite team.
- Whichever group is called has to retreat rather than give chase.

8. King of the Sea

Equipment: One bean bag per person, except the King or Queen

Skills: Gross motor skills, listening, attention

Imagery: The King (or Queen) of the Sea lives in a castle under the seas. Every day, ambassadors from every species of fish come to pay homage and seek the King's counsel, and sometimes they get invited to magnificent banquets. The fishes know that when the King invites them, they must quickly respond, or they will may not get the chance to enter the Banquet Hall.

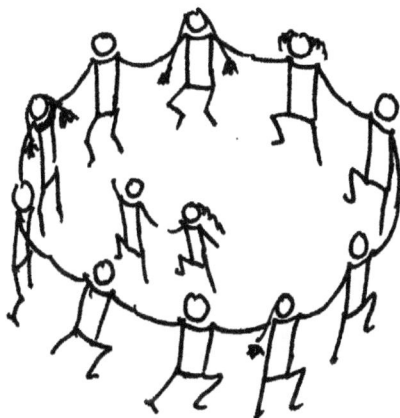

To play:
- Children sit in a big circle, facing in. Two children are the King (or Queen) standing in the middle. A bean bag marks the spot where each child sits.
- Each child chooses the name of a fish from a selection that the teacher gives (e.g. dolphin, shark, kingfisher, blue whale, flying fish).

- The King (or Queen) runs (or skip, hop, walk, etc.) around the inside of the circle, and calls out the name of a fish, e.g. Kingfisher:

  *"Kingfisher, Kingfisher, under the sea
  Kingfisher, Kingfisher, follow me"*

- This is the command for all the fishes so named to get up and follow the King (or Queen), running on the outside of the circle.

- The King or Queen takes their time and suddenly says *"Kingfisher, come dine with me!"*, and immediately sits in a vacant spot. The other fishes quickly follow and the two children who missed out on a seat become the next King (or Queen) of the Sea.

- The game may go on continuously and ends at the Teacher's discretion.

9. Copycat

Equipment: None

Skills: Gross motor, visual motor coordination

Imagery: Mama (or Papa) Cat needs to teach her kittens to follow instructions, but it is easier to teach them by showing them the right way to behave. Whatever Mama Cat does, the kittens imitate, but they have to do it without giving away Mama Cat's identity.

To play:
- One child is Mama or Papa Cat, one or two children are the Guessers, and the rest are Copycats.
- The Guesser is sent out of the room or has to close their eyes / shut their ears while the Teacher appoints Mama Cat.
- The children sit or stand in a circle, and the guesser is brought back in. Mama Cat initiates an action that the Copycats have to follow (such as pulling a funny face, stamping, clapping) while the guesser tries to discover the identity of Mama Cat.
- Whenever appropriate, Mama Cat switches the actions, and the Copycats have to follow without giving away Mama Cat's identity.
- If the guesser correctly guesses, the game is over, and new Mama Cat and guessers are chosen to start the game over.

10. Good Morning

Equipment: None

Skills: Spatial awareness, gross motor, listening, attention

Imagery: We have eyes to see and ears to hear. If we are attentive, our ears can tell us where sounds are coming from, even if we cannot see. The children in the Land of Mischief know this and they sometimes play tricks on their teacher. Someone would say 'Good Morning' when the teacher's back was to them and the poor teacher has to guess who it was who greeted them.

To play:
- This may be played in class or outdoors. One child is the Guesser and stands in front with their back to the rest of the class.
- The Teacher quietly selects someone as the Greeter, who has to greet the Guesser by their name, e.g. "Good Morning, Oliver".
- The Guesser, has to correctly identify the person (e.g. Natalie) who greeted them, by saying, "Good Morning, Natalie".
- If they guess correctly, they swap places. If not, swap them anyway, so everybody gets a chance, or give the Guesser three chances before choosing a new Guesser.

Variations:
- After greeting, give the class ten seconds to quietly move and change seats before the Guesser turns to face the class and tries to identify the Greeter.
- The game ends at the teacher's discretion.

11. Farmer, Farmer

Equipment: None

Skills: Gross motor, spatial awareness, agility, listening

Imagery: Children wish to play in the lush green meadows over the hills but must first request the farmer's permission to pass his farm. The farmer is grouchy and not pleased, so he plays a game of 'name the colour' with them.

To play:
- Children stand at one end of the play area. Two or more Farmers stand in the middle.
- The children sing:
  "Farmer, Farmer, may we pass. Over the hills and over the grass. If not, why not? What's your favourite colour? "
- Farmer calls a colour and any child with that colour visible tries to run safely to the other side without being tagged.
- If tagged, they turn into scarecrows on the spot, and help the Farmer tag children in the next round. They may not move their legs but may reach out with their hands.
- Once the first group makes it across, all others must follow. Repeat the process from the opposite side of the play area.
- Call *"Rainbow colours"*, and all have to run across.
- The game ends when there is a specific number of children left, then it is time to choose a new Farmer.

12. The Number Game

Equipment: None

Skills: Gross motor, spatial awareness, sensory awareness, number concept, agility, listening

Imagery: Once upon a time, there lived a sculptor, who loved numbers. Odd or even, they inspired his sculptures. When he needed inspiration he would close his eyes and imagine interesting shapes and patterns formed by combining numbers and body parts. Sometimes little children come to help him out.

To play:
- Teacher is the Sculptor who calls out instructions and children form groups to make interesting shapes as directed.
- For example, when the Teacher calls out "three children with six hands and four feet on the floor", the children huddle into groups of three to show their six hands, but only five feet on the floor. With six feet between them, they have to figure how to only have four feet on the floor. Perhaps two might stand on one foot each, or perhaps one might stand on another child's foot. Other examples:
    - four (children) with eight feet in the air
    - six (children) with five elbows touching
    - seven (children) with five mouths open
    - two hands, two feet and two heads
    - four bottoms and six hands
- There are no penalties and the odd child or children out may continue to join in for the next sculpture.

13. Please Mr Crocodile

Equipment: None

Skills: Gross motor, spatial awareness, agility, listening

Imagery: Children wish to cross the river to see Mr Crocodile's baby daughter. Mr Crocodile is very selective and only those who meet certain conditions are allowed through. Those who do not, risk being bitten by Mr Crocodile.

To play:
- Children stand at one end of the play area. Two or more crocodiles stand in the middle.
- The children sing:
  "Please Mr Crocodile, may we cross the river,
  To see your baby daughter?"
- Crocodile replies with something like "Yes, only if you are wearing blue" or "... if you have red hair".
- Those who meet the conditions may safely cross the river, after which all others must cross at their own peril, for Mr Crocodile will try to tag them.
- Tagged players become crocodiles and assist Mr Crocodile to tag the children in the next rounds.
- Repeat the process from the opposite side of the play area. The game ends when the crocodile has caught a specific number of children, or when there are a specified number of children left, then it is time to choose new Mr Crocodiles.

14. Come Play with Me[44]

Equipment: None

Skills: Gross motor, coordination, attention

Imagery: One day, the colour Yellow was feeling bright and cheerful and wanted someone to play with. It stretched out towards quiet and lonely Blue, who shied away. It flowed towards dynamic Red, who was too busy to notice. Yellow did not give up easily, and its cheerful disposition soon encouraged the other colours to come out to play. Perhaps, they might even create a rainbow in the sky!

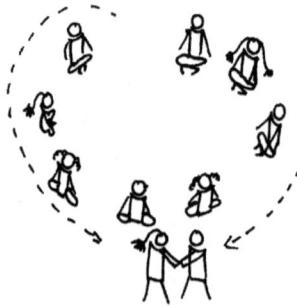

To play:
- The children pick a colour they'd like to be: Yellow, Red or Blue, and stand in a circle. One child is the colour Yellow who stands outside the circle and runs around, to touch someone on the back and say, "Come play with me!"
- The tagged colour runs in the opposite direction to catch up with the tagger, and on meeting, take hold of each other's hands (perhaps they can identify what colour have they created), swing once around, then race for the vacated spot.
- The first person back is safe, and the other becomes the new colour tagger.
- The game ends at the Teacher's discretion.

---

[44] The story is inspired by colour play and the game inspired by (Johnson, 1907)

15. Hunters, Hares and Hounds (1)[45]

Equipment: One ball

Skills: Gross motor, spatial awareness, agility, ball handling skills

Imagery: It's early in the morning and hunters have gathered to go hare hunting. Because of the dense cover and gnarly tangles of briar, thorns and honeysuckle, they have brought their trusty Hound to trail after hares. All are dreaming of stewed hare at the end of the day.

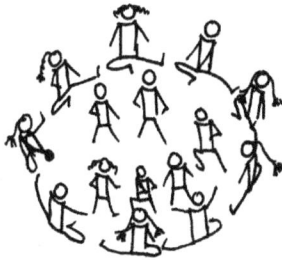

To play:
- One group of children are the Hunters, sitting in a circle, facing in, with legs wide out. The other group are the Hares, standing in the middle.
- One Hunter begins by rolling the ball (the Hound) along the ground to tag the legs of a Hare in the middle. Hares try to dodge the Hound.
- The tagged Hare collects the ball and swaps places with the Hunter who tagged it.
- Encourage the children not to hold on to the ball too long, so I usually have a 5 second rule.

Variations:
- Add an extra ball

---

45   This is the simplest version: circle formation, ball roll and tagged child replaces the tagger.

16. Cat and Mouse (1)[46]

Equipment: None

Skills: Gross motor, spatial awareness, agility, teamwork

Imagery: A long, long, time ago, the Jade Emperor announced a race! The first twelve animals to make it across the river would be rewarded with a year named in their honour in the Chinese Zodiac[47] calendar. All the animals were excited, and none more so than Cat and Mouse, who were very good friends. The Cat decided it would be wise to take a nap before the big race, and Mouse promised to wake him up in time.

However, the cunning Mouse did not keep his promise to the Cat. Instead, he persuaded the burly Ox to let him ride on his broad back across the river because he could not swim. Then he tricked the Ox by jumping off Ox's back as they neared shore, and in so doing, was named the first animal of the zodiac. The other animals came next, but not poor Cat who was still asleep. When Cat woke up, he was devastated and furious. Since that time, Cats and Mice have never been friends.

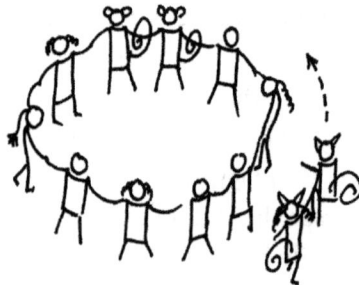

---

[46] There are many versions of Cat and Mouse, and this is suitable for younger children. It is less confronting, less spatially demanding and the child has the group's protection.

[47] Story is based on the Chinese Zodiac Story.

To play:

- The children form a circle, facing in and holding hands. One pair among them is chosen to be the Mouse. Standing outside this circle is the Cat (another pair of children holding hands).
- The Cat tries to catch the designated Mouse, but the Mouse runs away, by moving with his 'house' – the rest of the circle, who may rotate to protect the Mouse from being caught.
- The game ends when the Mouse is caught, and a new pair of Cat and Mouse is chosen.
- If the chase drags on, consider appointing a new Cat, Mouse, or both.
- To help keep the circle shape, consider having a point of reference in the middle of the circle (e.g. teacher standing in the middle, placing cones, or marking a circle on the ground), reminding the children that the circle they form must be within the designated boundary.

17. Shooting Star

Equipment: None

Skills: Gross motor, midline crossing, bilateral integration, spatial awareness, coordination

Imagery: Once upon a time, the Man on the Moon went for a ride on a Shooting Star and tumbled down to Earth. There he stayed and played with the children, and waited for the next Shooting Star shuttle to take him and some children back to the Moon. But they must be quick to catch the tail of the Shooting Star before the sparks fizzle out.

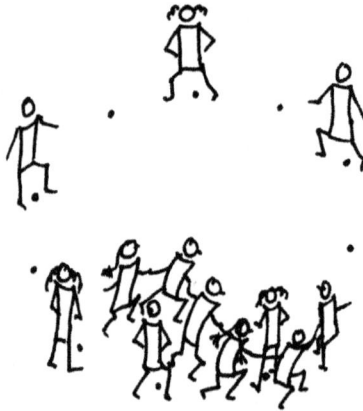

To play: • One child is the Man on the Moon, and one child is the Shooting Star. All others are children who wish to go for a ride to the Moon.

• The children stand in a big circle, facing in. The Shooting Star leads the Man on the Moon by the hand and they weave in and out of the circle. They make a few stops, anywhere in the circle, each time picking up a child to join them on the journey to the moon. Each child joins the chain tag, until there are eight to ten children in the chain.

- The chain is joined by children holding hands, but with a cross-over. For example, Shooting Star uses his right hand to clasp Man on the Moon's left hand. Man on the Moon uses his right hand to hold on to the first child's left hand, and the first child uses his right hand to hold on to the second child's left hand, and so on.
- When there are eight to ten people in the chain, the two ends of the chain join hands, facing in. At a signal, they pull and break the chain that will send them tumbling down onto the moon.
- The game may be repeated with new students taking on the role of the Man on the Moon and the Shooting Star. Try to give every child a chance to be in the chain.

18. Obstacle Course

Equipment: Cones, gym mats, climbing frame, crawling tunnels, benches, balance beams, bean bags, ground markers, hula hoops, scooter boards, balls, etc.

Skills: Gross motor skills, hand-eye coordination, core muscle strength development, throwing skills, balancing skills

Imagery: Once upon a time, there lived a wise Queen who ruled over a land where everyone was happy, kind and smiling. One day, the Queen noticed several sad faces in her kingdom, and yet more the next day. Her knights discovered that some mischievous goblins have been stealing the happy smiles. So she sent her knights on a mission to find the thieves and recover the smiles before her land became a land of gloom. Her knights need all the help they can get. Who is ready to go on this quest to help the Queen?

To play:
- Set up an obstacle course using whatever props are available and appropriate for the story, or make up your own.
- Incorporate developmental exercises, activities that develop core muscle strength, gross motor skills, eye-hand coordination (for example rolling, crawling, tunnelling, climbing, walking on balance beam, throwing, catching, skipping, etc.) and finishing with a collection of objects they have to retrieve for the Queen, in this case the Smiles, such as bean bags tossed into a basket, or retrieving objects in a sensory bag.
- Demonstrate how to navigate the course and what the objective is.
- Students stand in a row and one at a time, they set off on the quest, ensuring a smooth flow.

- Students may only step on designated safe areas of the course. Stepping off the course will send them to 'hospital' (i.e. return to the start line).
- Incorporate as many obstacles or danger zones as is appropriate.
- Students who have completed the obstacle and retrieved an object of the quest may begin the quest again.
- The game may go on, and ends at the teacher's discretion.

Year Two: (Ages 7 - 8)
Developmental Picture of the Eight-Year-Old:
Awakening

The eight-year-old, it seems, has woken up from the dreamy state to awe at the world before them. The energies that were used to form the physical body is now freed to work on the rhythmic or feeling realm. Awakened like a butterfly from its cocoon, the child dances and prances on the currents of wonder, joy, pity, tenderness and sorrow[48] to find their relationship to the world around them.

The child is more energetic, lively, dexterous, physically confident, individualistic and eager for more challenges. Their ability to concentrate and focus is stronger, and they seem to have an opinion about everything. They are very open, trusting, and still live in a vivid world of imagination. They resonate strongly with the stories of fables and legends, and recognise the everyday attributes of humans as shown through animals. These feeling qualities appeal to them and the saintly qualities are something they can strive for.

---

[48] Manette Teitlbaum (in Dendtler, 2018)

Movement Emphasis for Year 2

- Developing gross and fine motor abilities and spatial awareness.
- Games continue to involve the use of imagination, embodying the moral qualities portrayed in fables and legends; games that explore polarities of good and evil; games that convey courage and endurance (e.g. knights and dragons) and games that encourage cooperation, tolerance and sharing.
- Games should have an archetypal character, song/rhyme and movement.
- The teacher is encouraged to be the protagonist, otherwise, have two or more take on the role of the protagonist.

The Teacher's Sheath of Authority:

The Saint

The Year Two teacher conveys wisdom and benevolent kindness, working out of the image of the Saint[49] – wise, all-knowing, with an authority that stems from good intentions: "Do what I say because I know what is best." Whether it is 'No hat, no play' 'No work, no play'– that is the rule; follow it because I know what is best.

The Saint also inspires the students to do what is good, noble and true as an act of kindness, gently correcting any misdemeanour.

---

[49] Dan Freeman (personal communication)

1. Zip, Zap, Pass the Clap

Equipment: None

Skills: Midline crossing, rhythm, attention, focus, coordination

Imagery: High up in the clouds, the King of Thunder wanted to teach his children how to handle the thunderbolt. So he bade them gather and sealed the energy into the palm of his hands and sent it off to each and every child in turn to practice.

To play:
- All players stand in a circle, facing inwards. Teacher is the King of Thunder, who begins by sending a clap towards the person next to them.
- The second person responds by quickly passing the clap onwards to the next person. The third person does the same until the clap is passed all around and comes back to the Teacher.

Variations:
- When students get better, go faster or follow with their chest or other parts of their body.
- For older children, instead of always passing the clap in the same direction, they may choose to reverse the direction of the clap. When this is played, remind students to ensure that others in the circle get a chance to receive and pass the clap.
- For much older children (Year 6 onwards) they may also redirect the clap to someone across the circle.

2. Mouse / Possum Run

Equipment: None

Skills: Synchronicity, eye-hand coordination, attention

Imagery: I have a little mouse in my pocket who needs to do his daily exercise. He is also shy and dislikes loud noise. Shhhhh! He loves to run around in a circle and when I release him, please jump over the mouse one foot at a time when he comes your way. Remember to wait till he has come to you, for we do not want to jump on him!

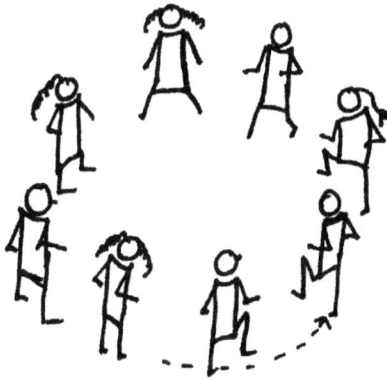

To play:
- Children stand in a circle, facing inward.
- Teacher takes imaginary mouse out of their pocket, places it on the ground, letting it run around the circle in one direction. Each child takes turns to jump over the mouse when it reaches them.
- Teacher catches the mouse when it returns after making a circuit around the class.
- Release the mouse in the other direction.

Variations: • Release a second mouse.
   • Instead of a mouse, release a possum[50], who has gotten loose in the wattle grove. This time, children raise hands high above their head and clap when the possum reaches them.

---

[50] A game first played with (Hungerford)

3. Dead Ant Tag

Equipment: Two sashes, several carpet squares or place markers

Skills: Gross motor, spatial awareness, body awareness, dodging skills

Imagery: Farmer Brown has a lovely strawberry patch that sometimes gets infected by ants. But he doesn't like to use any toxic spray, so he catches them one at a time, and leaves them for dead. However, the ants are only injured, and when they recover, they come back to the strawberry patch.

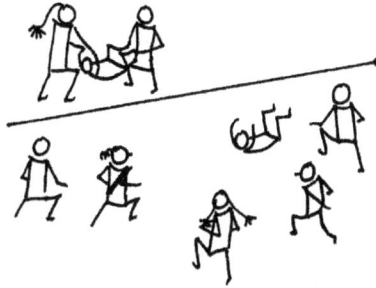

To play:
- Two children are Farmer Brown, all others are Ants.
- Place several carpet squares as 'Ant's Nests' where ants are safe from being tagged. Each nest holds two or three ants (depending on its size). Ants may not stay home for more than 5 seconds.
- Farmer Brown chases and tags the ants. Tagged ants lay on the ground with legs and arms waving about in the air. They are rescued by four ants, each holding on to a limb, dragging them out of the boundary, where they immediately recover and are able to re-join the game. Ants cannot be tagged when they are rescuing.
- The game ends after a specified time, to allow for a swap of roles.

4. Frogs on the Lily Pads

Equipment: Two sashes, hula hoops, spot marker

Skills: Gross motor, spatial awareness, body awareness

Imagery: Down by the banks of the river, live an army of frogs who love to gather and chat about their favourite meal, when they are not off catching flies, wriggly worms, slugs or snails. One day, while they were sitting on their lily pads discussing snails and slugs, and other yummy food, a goanna comes by looking for his lunch!

To play:
- Scatter several hula hoops (lily pads) around the play area, and one sport marker for Goanna's lunch box.
- Two children (with sashes) are the Goannas, who make "Hisss" sounds but when they catch a frog, they go "Slurp". All others are Frogs who go "Ribbit".
- Frogs run (or hop) around catching insects and avoid being caught by the Goannas. They are only safe when on a lily pad.
- Each lily pad may hold one frog at any time for 5 seconds, otherwise the lily pad will sink.
- When a Frog is caught, they go into the Goanna's lunch box. However, there is a hole in the lunch box, and when the fifth frog gets thrown in, the first frog escapes.
- The game goes on endlessly, and the teacher can call a halt and change Goannas.

5. Hunters, Hares and Hounds (2)[51]

Equipment: A soft dodge ball

Skills: Gross motor, ball handling skills, spatial awareness

Imagery: It's early in the morning and hunters have gathered to go hare hunting. Because of the dense cover and gnarly tangles of briar, thorns and honeysuckle, they have brought their trusty Hound to trail after hares. All are dreaming of stewed hare at the end of the day.

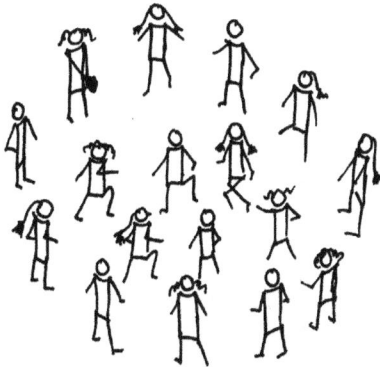

To play:
- One group or children are the Hunters, and they form a circle surrounding a smaller group standing within (the Hares).
- Teacher or a Hunter starts by throwing a ball (Hound) underarm, to tag the legs of a Hare in the middle (from the knees down).
- A tagged Hare collects the ball and swaps places with the tagger.

---

51 This version: in circle formation, underarm toss, tagged child replaces the tagger.

99

Variation: • Add an extra ball.

• All children are Hares standing in the middle, except one child who is the Hunter standing in the outer circle. The Hunter aims to tag a Hare (knees down). A tagged Hare joins the Hunting team with no replacement. The objective is to get all players in the middle out (see Hunters, Hares and Hounds (3)).

6. Bird Catcher

Equipment: Scarves or sashes in red, yellow, blue and green, one for each child (or other appropriate colours)

Skills: Gross motor, listening, attention, concentration

Imagery: Deep in the forest, live many species of exotic birds who thrill so beautifully that their songs could be heard for miles. This attracts a bird catcher! One day, while the little fledglings are out learning to hunt, Mother bird spies a bird catcher, and cries out in alarm for the birds to return.

To play:
- Teacher is Mother Bird, who stands at one end of the play area (the nest), two or more children are Bird Catchers, who stand in the middle, and all others are birds, at the other end (the forest). Designate an area as the bird cage.
- Children are divided into four groups of birds identified by their colours (green for parrots, red for robins, blue for bluebird, and yellow for canary).
- Mother Bird calls out a type of bird to return, and those so assigned have to flap their wings and run back to the nest. A bird is safe if it reaches the nest, but if they are caught, they go to the bird cage.
- Mother bird calls for the next group, and play is repeated until all groups have had a run. When all have had a go, open the bird cage and choose new Mother Bird and Bird Catchers.

Variation:
- Call for more than one group at a time.
- Have a Daddy Bird who rescues the birds from the bird cage, so they can return to the forest. Daddy bird is safe from the bird catcher.

7. Three Billy Goats Gruff

Equipment: Two sashes

Skills: Core muscle strength, attention and coordination

Imagery: The mean and ugly troll lives under the bridge. He waits for unsuspecting billy goats to trip trap across and catches them for lunch. He stuffs the first goat into his lunch box, and another, and another, but his lunch box never gets full, because the goats have learnt to outwit him!

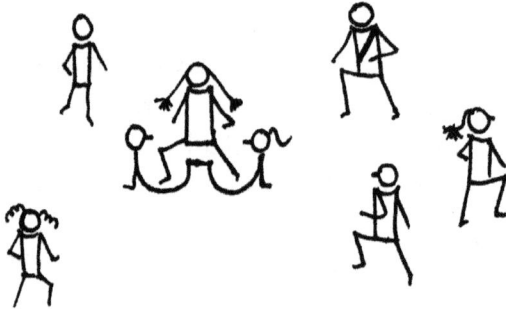

To play:
- Two or more children are Trolls and the rest are Goats.
- The Troll begins by chasing and trying to tag the Goats. When Goats are tagged, they sit down on the spot, on their bottoms with knees bent and feet raised so that the lower legs are parallel to the ground – forming part of a bridge. Two Goats may join to form a bridge.
- A third Goat saves the pair by jumping over the bridge. The play goes on endlessly, until the Teacher calls for a change of Troll.

8. Sheep in the Stable

Equipment: None

Skills: Gross motor, spatial awareness and orientation, quick reaction, agility, listening

Imagery: Sheep graze in the paddocks and at nightfall have to find their way into nice warm stables, but there are not enough stables, and one or two sheep are always left shivering for the night. Brrrrgh! So when they hear the Shepherd call "Sheep in Stables", they run quickly into the stables.

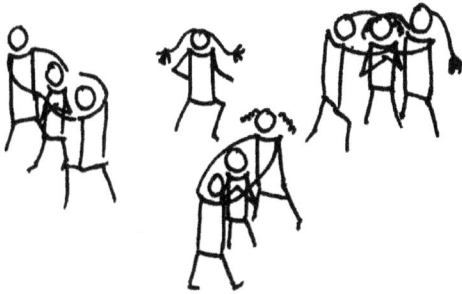

To play:
- Children in groups of three, scattered around the play area.
- Two players in each group hold hands to form a stable, and the third stands in the middle. One or two sheep have no stable.
- When the teacher says, "Sheep in the paddock!", all the sheep come out and run around the paddock. When the teacher says, "Sheep in the stables!", all the sheep have to find a stable.
- Each stable may only hold one sheep, and the odd sheep or two is homeless for the night and stands shivering. As soon

as the stable is full, the game is repeated. Sheep may not enter the same stable they were just in.

- Ensure sheep and stables swap roles so everyone has a chance to be a sheep.

Variations:
- Call "Sheep to Stables" and the sheep change stables. Call "Stables to Sheep", and the Sheep stay put and Stables have to find a new partner to form a stable, and a new sheep to house. They may not form a stable with their previous partners.
- Instead of Sheep and Stables, the children are Squirrels and Trees. Use commands like: Squirrels out and about / Squirrels up a tree / Squirrels Change /Trees Change!
- Other images to use are Hares and Hounds, Koalas and Dingos, the choice is endless.

9. Shark, Seaweed and Rocks

Equipment: None

Skills: Spatial awareness, gross motor, listening, attention, agility

Imagery: Schools of fish are trying to swim across a shark infested reef. The sharks demand a token – fish of a certain colour. The fishes comply by sending their bravest to challenge the shark in order to confuse him. When the sharks are preoccupied, the rest of the fishes try to swim across.

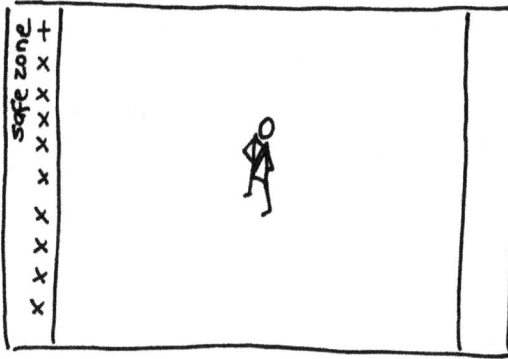

To play:
- Set up the play area with two boundary lines at opposite ends of the play area. This is the safe zone. All the Fishes start at one of these ends, and the Shark or Sharks stand in the middle
- The Shark(s) call out a colour. Fishes with that colour visible have to brave the Shark by being the first to swim across the reef to safety. When this group of fish make it across, the rest of the Fishes then follow.
- The Shark(s) try to tag the Fishes as they swim by. Tagged Fishes stay put on the spot where they are tagged and become seaweed.

- A Seaweed helps the Shark to tangle the Fish as they swim by. They stand astride with arms by their sides to tangle the Fish as they run past. When the Seaweed touches a Fish, that Fish becomes a Seaweed as well.
- The game ends when a specified number of Fishes are left, who may become the next Sharks.

Variation:
- Tagged Fishes can choose to become Rocks, in which case they stand with their legs crossed and their arms across their chest. These Rocks are fish friendly and give shelter for the Fish to hide from the Sharks.
- Sharks may call "Rainbow colours" and all the Fishes have to run across at the same time.
- As above, but all Fishes and Sharks are in pairs. When each Fish pair is tagged by the Shark pair, they become Rocks. If the Shark pair breaks the chain, all the Rocks are free.

10. Cat and Mouse (2)[52]

Equipment: None

Skills: Spatial awareness, agility, quick reaction, cooperation

Imagery: Cat and Mouse were once very good friends, but they had a falling out. The Cat accuses the Mouse of being cunning and the Mouse accuses the Cat of being lazy. And now whenever they meet, tensions flare! (For the full story, see Cat and Mouse (1)).

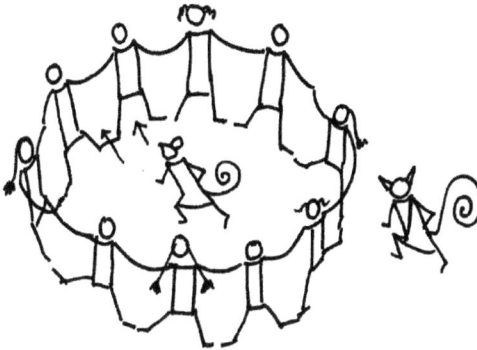

To play:
- One child is the Cat and another is the Mouse. All others stand astride in a circle, holding hands, adjacent feet touching.
- Mouse starts inside the circle and the Cat from outside trying to catch the Mouse.
- Both Cat and Mouse may run through the open windows (legs), but the circle assists the Mouse by raising their

---

[52] Moving on from the Mouse House version in Class 1, this is the Windows and Doors version, where the Mouse still has some protection from the group, but it is more spatially demanding as there is movement from outside the circle to the inside and from the centre to the outside.

clasped hands to help the Mouse move in and out easily, and lowering their hands to prevent the Cat from following.

- The game ends when the Mouse is caught, and a new pair of Cat and Mouse is chosen.
- Relieve slow exhausted or indifferent runners by nominating a new pair of Cat and Mouse.
- If the chase drags on, consider opening doors (circle drop hands) to allow the Cat a chance to catch the Mouse.

Variations:
- Consider a Cat and Mouse pair. If children are still anxious of being confronted by a protagonist, pair an insecure child with a more secure child.
- With a large group of children, consider having two or more Cat and Mice (identified with sashes).
- If children are ready, swap roles when the Mouse is caught: the caught Mouse becomes the new Cat, and the chasing Cat becomes the new Mouse.

11. Dingo and Possum

Equipment: Two or three beanbags of different colours

Skills: Crossing midline, eye-hand coordination, rhythm, concentration, throwing and catching, quick reaction

Imagery: A possum is out in the forest foraging for food, and guess who has picked up his scent? A very hungry dingo who sneaks up quietly. Can he catch up to the possum?

To play:
- All sit or stand in a circle, facing in. Designate one beanbag as the Possum and the other, Dingo.
- The objective is for the Dingo to catch the Possum.
- Teacher begins by passing Possum to the right or left, and children pass it along quickly without holding on or dropping it.
- When Possum is halfway around the circle, the Teacher releases the Dingo (a different coloured bean bag). Depending on how close the Dingo is, the Possum may run faster, or may change directions and run the other way. The Dingo may do likewise in pursuit.
- The game ends when the Dingo catches the Possum.

Variation:
- If the Possum is too quick, add another Dingo.
- For much older children, the Dingo may even be thrown across the circle in pursuit, and the Possum may do likewise.

12. Bunnies and Burrows

Equipment: Four to five hula hoops, two sashes

Skills: Gross motor, spatial awareness, agility

Imagery: Bunnies have made their burrows in the farmer's lettuce garden and usually come out for breakfast at the break of dawn. The Fox knows this, and he has come out from his den and hides in waiting!

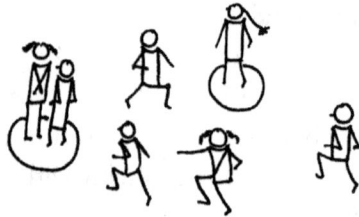

To play:
- Scatter hula hoops (burrows) around the play area.
- Two children are chosen as the Foxes (wearing sashes) who start at one end of the play area (their den) and all others are Bunnies, hopping around.
- On the Teacher's signal, the Foxes start to chase the Bunnies.
- Bunnies run for safety, but the burrows are small and can only fit three Bunnies at any time, and each can only stay in there for no more than 5 seconds. When a new Bunny comes in, one Bunny has to hop out, usually the one who has been in there the longest.
- A tagged Bunny goes into the Fox's lunch box in the den, which can only fit three Bunnies. The fourth one squeezed in pushes the first one out.
- The game can go on endlessly, and Teacher can halt the game occasionally to choose new foxes.

13. Flea Catcher

Equipment: None

Skills: Sensory and spatial awareness, gross motor, agility

Imagery: It is flea season and the fleas are everywhere, on hair, clothes, ears, beards and armpits. Fleas bite and makes you itch! If someone gets bitten too many times, they need the Flea Catcher!

To play:
- All children are Fleas ready to infect everyone else, by chasing each other, and one child is the Flea Catcher, who stays in a designated spot.
- When tagged, players place one hand on the spot on their body where they were tagged and pretend to scratch as if it itches. They can continue to tag others with their free hand.
- If they are tagged a second time, they place their other hand on the spot and start scratching. They are now unable to tag others but may run around to avoid being tagged a third time.
- If tagged a third time, they have to go to the Flea Catcher who gently taps them on the shoulder and they are cured. If demand for the Flea Catcher's service is high, they may have to stand in line and wait their turn.
- Once cured, they re-join the game. The game goes on endlessly until the Teacher calls for a change of Flea Catcher.

14. Ha! Ha! Ha!

Equipment: None

Skills: Sensory awareness, humour

Imagery: Once upon a time, there was a mischievous Elf who ran into a classroom of hardworking children to play tricks on them. First, he sprinkles a sleeping powder over them, sending them into deep sleep, huddled up together. All is quiet and calm. Then he wakes them up with another sprinkle of Elfin powder, and all they can say upon waking is 'Ha'.

To play:
- Children form circles of six to eight, or in a long line. The first child lies on their back on the ground and each subsequent child lies with their head on the tummy of the child before, in a zig zag formation. If possible, close the loop, so the first child's head is resting on the tummy of the last child.
- The first child says "Ha" while trying to maintain a straight face. The next child says "Ha! Ha!" and the third child says "Ha! Ha! Ha!" and so on. It doesn't take long before they are all laughing hysterically.
- How long can they stay calm?

15. Big Bear

Equipment: None

Skills: Gross motor, coordination, spatial awareness, balance

Imagery: Big Bear is hungry and is hunting for some plump, juicy children for lunch. But he is also old and short-sighted, so the children trick him by pretending to be trees and keeping very still. Big Bear sniffs and goes away confused. Tagged children go into the Bear's lunch box, but his lunch box has only space for three children and the fourth child caught pushes the first child out!

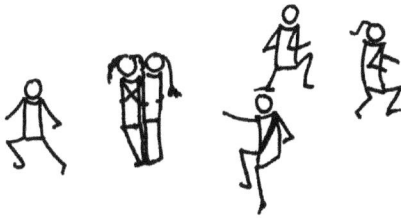

To play:
- Two children are Big Bear, identified by their sashes. Mark a place for the bear's lunch box.
- Big Bear gives chase, and tagged children go to his lunch-box. They re-join the game when they get pushed out of the lunch box.
- Children can avoid being tagged by coming together as a pair and pretending to be a tree: one person in the pair has to have their feet off the ground (piggyback or stepping on partner's toes).
- The game goes on until the Teacher calls for a change of Big Bear.

Variations:
- Vary the number of children in the lunch box.

16. House on Wheels

Equipment: Bean bags or place markers for each pair of children

Skills: Gross motor, agility, spatial awareness

Imagery: Once upon a time, there was a Little House on wheels, who didn't have a permanent home. One day, it came to an enchanted glade where it met other little houses on wheels. Some were parked where they had a view of the mountain, or river, or the waterfall, and they were all happy to share and trade places with Little House, so it could get a view.

To play:
- The children stand (or sit) in pairs, in a circle, with one pair (Little House) standing in the middle. Each pair is a House, and each House is numbered 1, 2, 3, etc. Place a bean bag on the ground to mark the spot where each House stands.
- Little House calls out two numbers to exchange places, while it tries to get to one of the vacated spots. The House that fails to get a spot, becomes the next Little House.
- If Little House calls out "House on Wheels", all houses have to exchange places, but not with the House immediately to their right or left. Little House tries to get into one of the vacated spots.
- Each pair runs with hands linked. The pair that breaks the link becomes the new Little House.
- The game can go one continuously and ends at the Teacher's discretion.

17. Wolf in Sheep's Clothing[53]

Equipment: A sash for each Wolf (and one for each Shepherd)

Skills: Gross motor, agility spatial awareness

Imagery: Every morning when the Sheep are let out onto the paddocks, they do their happy dance, for they are glad that Mr Wolf is nowhere to be seen. Little do they know that he is hiding among them, disguised as a Sheep!

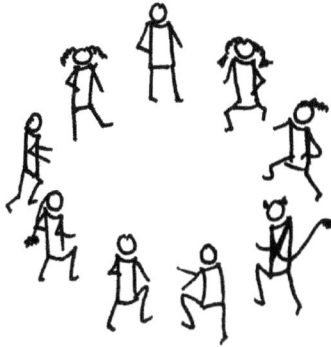

To play:
- The children are all Sheep, standing in a circle, facing outwards. In the circle is a coloured sash.
- The teacher quietly walks around the inside of the circle, whispering in the ear of a few students. To a few of them, whisper "Mr / Mrs Wolf" and they are the designated the Wolf in Sheep's clothing.
- To start, the children turn to face inwards, and skip around in a circle, chanting:
  "The morning has dawned. The wolf is gone.
  He isn't here, he isn't there. He isn't anywhere!"

---

[53] This game is adapted from van Haren & Kischnick (1999)

- Chant the verse once in its entirety. Anytime during the second chant, Mr Wolf suddenly throws off his disguise, and announces his intention to give chase, by running into the circle, picking up and putting on the sash.
- Tagged Sheep go into the Wolf's lunch box (which can hold four or more Sheep) and await rescue (e.g. when the fifth Sheep comes in, the first Sheep goes out). This game goes on and on until the Teacher calls for a change of Wolf, and the game starts all over again.

Variations:
- When the Wolf has caught a certain number of Sheep, the game restarts.
- Introduce the Shepherd who knows how sneaky the Wolf can be and also hides among the sheep. When the Wolf reveals himself and starts chasing the sheep, the Shepherd comes to the rescue (in this case, place a sash of a different colour in the middle of the circle). The Shepherd can rescue one Sheep at a time by pulling them out of the lunch box and into a safe zone before going back to rescue another).

18. Earth, Air, Water, Fire[54]

Equipment: A soft foam ball or bean bag, marker for fire pit

Skills: Listening, memory, alertness, ball handling skills

Imagery: A long, long, time ago, Mother Earth and Father Sun, Sister Rain and Brother Wind had a conversation about how they would like to give a little of themselves to make the world a beautiful place. So Father Sun offered fire to give warmth to the cold earth so it could sustain life on earth, Mother Earth gave minerals, plant and animal life on land, Sister Rain gave water and life to animals who live in it, and Brother Wind gave air for all to breath and animals who could soar in the sky. Can you name any of these animals?

To play:
- Children stand in a circle. The Teacher stands in the middle with a ball or bean bag. The Teacher begins by throwing a ball to a child while calling out for example, "Earth".
- The child addressed has to catch the ball and name an animal that lives on land, for example 'Cat', then throws the ball back to the Teacher.
- If the Teacher says "Air", the catcher has to name a bird; if 'Water', they name a fish. If 'Fire', they may not catch the ball, but let it fall to the ground.
- Children are sent to the Fire Pit if they catch the ball on 'Fire', repeat an answer already given, take too long to reply (five seconds or more) or fail to give an answer. The Fire Pit has space for three children, and the fourth child in sends the first child out to re-join the game.

---

[54] A story inspired by a game from (Greenaway, 1889) and (Squareman, 1916)

Year Three (Ages 8 - 9)

Developmental Picture of the Nine-Year-Old:

Rubicon Crossing

This is a developmentally significant year for the nine-year-old child. They stand in the middle, between the world of early childhood and the world of adolescence. They are given a glimpse of what lies beyond and start to face numerous physical and emotional challenges. The child may have a growth spurt and their physical proportions changes. They are more active, coordinated and skilful. Cognitively more capable, the child's concentration is stronger and their ability for self-directed exploration increases.

The nine-year-old is also a paragon of contradictions, with conflicting emotions – moody one minute, fine the next. They could be increasingly self-assured in some ways, yet anxious and insecure in others. They may start to question their origins and destiny, and about birth and death. Socially, they seek increasing independence, yet could need to seek refuge within the family.

They are more aware of the world around them and relate to the world from a new perspective. This period is often referred to as the crossing of the Rubicon[55], the crossing of the river of consciousness, the point of no return to the dreamy innocence of childhood.

---

[55] In ancient times, the river Rubicon marked the border between the heart of Rome and the Roman province of Gaul. To cross this border was a declaration of war. In 49 BCE, Julius Caesar, on returning from his conquest of Gaul, did just that, starting a war against Pompey and the Roman Senate. This phrase is now synonymous with committing to a cause of action which may bring great changes and significant risks.

Movement Emphasis for Year 3

- The emphasis is on developing physical dexterity, spatial orientation, co-ordination, rhythm and concentration.
- Games where obstacles are experienced, and which explore mental powers, attention, observation, imagination, reasoning, memory, rhythm and values.
- Games that allow the class to experience challenges as a collective 'we', and then to start building independence from this collective group soul.
- Games and movement that encourage an inner discipline and an inner stillness. To be willing to do one's part in the team and to see the outer world with a growing awareness of their inner world, so that this may translate into the ability for self-direction and purpose in life.
- The flexibility and aliveness brought about through movement will translate into their thinking.

The Teacher's Sheath of Authority:

The Patriarch / Matriarch

The nine-year-old child is awakening to the world around them. They need to have the room to expand and experience this new awareness, while being held by the security and authority of the Teacher, in a clear and consistent manner, and provided with the curriculum to meet those needs. The child is seeking reassurance that the authority of the Teacher carries with it an inner certainty.

The image of authority for this age is that of the Patriarch / Matriarch[56], one of absolute law – this is how it is, because I said so. This is the rule of my house. Rules are black and white.

---

[56] Dan Freeman (personal communication)

1. Accidents

Equipment: Two sashes, one to three coloured markers

Skills: Spatial awareness, gross motor, agility, cooperation

Imagery: Who has had an accident? Ouch! Accidents happen anywhere and anytime! They creep up on us when we are not careful, so it is important to stay mindful and alert. If you are caught by an accident, you will need an ambulance to take you to hospital. We must also help take our friends to hospital.

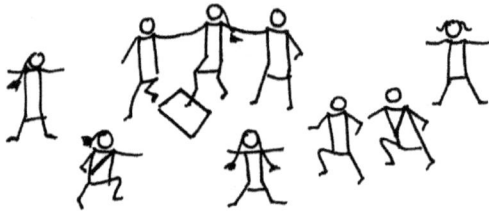

To play:
- Place coloured markers on the floor to represent Hospitals.
- Two or three children are the Accidents just waiting to happen, who chase and tag children.
- Tagged children stand on the spot, put their hands out by their sides, and wait for an Ambulance.
- An Ambulance consists of two drivers, one on either side of the victim, holding their hands and taking them to Hospital. As soon as the victim steps into Hospital, they immediately recover. Players are safe from tagging when linked.
- Accidents may not 'puppy guard' a Hospital.
- The game goes on until the Teacher calls for new Accidents or until all children are caught and there are no Ambulance drivers left.

2. Candlestick Tag

Equipment: Two or more sashes

Skills: Spatial awareness, gross motor, cooperation

Imagery: Once upon a time, there lived a Witch in the Enchanted Forest who has bewitched her garden to produce the most delicious blueberries, raspberries, strawberries and many other kinds of berries. Now, Pixies are always sneaking into her garden to feast on them. This annoys the Witch, so she casts a magic spell to turn the Pixies into Candlesticks. She places these Candlesticks on her windowsill as a warning to other pixies. However, the mischievous Pixies learn how to free their friends.

To play:
- One or two children are the Witch or Wizard (identified by sash). All others are Pixies.
- The Witch chases and tags the Pixies, turning them into Candlesticks (stand astride, arms above head and palms together).
- Clever Pixies save their friends by crawling between their legs. While crawling through, they are safe from the Witch's magic spell.

Variations:
- Instead of Witches, it is the Farmers protecting their crop of corn from the crows and they cast a spell to turn the crows into Scarecrows. They stand with their arm wide at chest level.

3. Monkeys and Bananas

Equipment: Four sashes of two different colours

Skills: Dodging, gross motor, agility

Imagery: It is banana harvest time, but a big storm is blowing all the bananas away. The Farmer runs around trying to put a net over the bananas. However, the sneaky Monkeys see their chance, and swoop in for a feast.

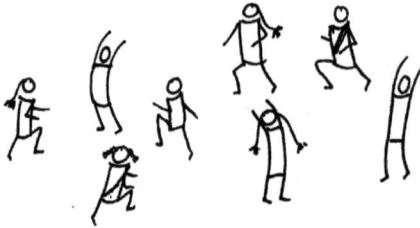

To play:
- Two children are Farmers (with sashes), and two are Monkeys (different coloured sashes). All others are Bananas, who scatter as if blown away by the wind.
- Farmers tag flyaway Bananas who freeze on the spot with their hands above their head, leaning to one side in the shape of a banana.
- Along come two Monkeys, one on either side pulling the Banana's arms down, as if peeling a banana skin off. Once a Banana's skin is peeled off, they can re-join the game.
- This game goes on endlessly and the Teacher can call for a change of Farmer and Monkeys.

Variations:
- Bananas that get peeled and eaten by Monkeys go to the Greenhouse and wait to re-join the game. The Greenhouse has space for four Bananas and the fifth one coming in pushes the first one out.

4. Wildfire

Equipment: Two or more sashes

Skills: Spatial awareness, gross motor, cooperation

Imagery: A fire is a good friend but a very bad enemy. They keep us warm, but when not contained, they can spread and cause a lot of damage. Two little Fire Sparks are being blown about by the wind and they are spreading their sparks wherever they go. How long will it be before the whole place is up in smoke?

To play:
- One or two children are the Fire Sparks and all others are children running away from them.
- The Fire Sparks chase and tag the children. Both ends of the Fire Spark may tag, and tagged children join the Fire Spark chain.
- Whenever the chain becomes four, they split into two groups of two, and the tagging continues.
- The game ends when all the children have been tagged.

5. Tit for Tat

Equipment: None

Skills: Spatial awareness, gross motor, agility

Imagery: Two hungry dingoes were out hunting one day. The first dingo caught a rabbit but refused to share its meal, so the second dingo bit it in the leg and sulked away. The next day, while they were out hunting, Second Dingo caught a large rabbit, and it too refused share its meal. So First Dingo bit it in the shoulder and sulked away. This tit for tat biting and hitting continued till both were too injured to hunt for food and had to starve till they recovered from their wounds.

To play:
- Children pair off, one is the First Dingo, and the other, the Second Dingo.
- First Dingo pursues Second Dingo. When tagged, Second Dingo turns around on the spot before pursuing First Dingo (giving it time to escape) and play continues in a tit for tat manner.
- Pairs 'Tit for Tat' tag each other only, without making physical contact with any other pairs. If they physically touch another person other than their partner, they must stop to shake hands with that person before continuing to evade or pursue their partner.

Variations:
- Begin with walking only, then include other variations, such as skipping, hopping on one leg or running.

6. Ship Ahoy!

Equipment: None

Skills: Spatial awareness, balance, agility, gross motor, courage

Imagery: The children are sailors, standing on shore and are trying to get back to their ship. Standing in their way is the fearsome Pegged Legged Pirate who wants to kidnap them for his pirate ship. He doesn't give them much of a choice, as he challenges them to 'Walk the Plank!' or 'Join the Crew!'

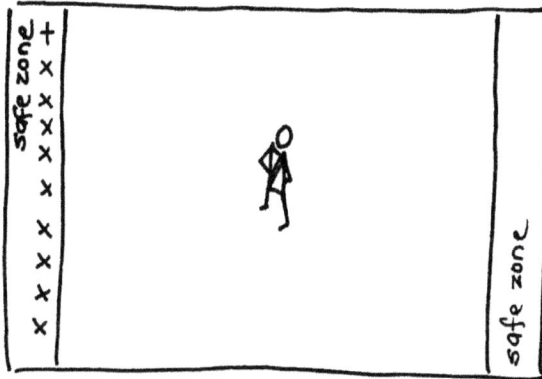

To play:
- The children stand at one end of the play area (shore) facing the opposite end (ship). One or two children are The Pegged Legged Pirate (hopping on one foot) who stand in their way.
- The sailors cry *"Pirates! Pirates! You can't catch me!"* The pirate calls a child by their name and challenges them to: *"Walk the plank or join the crew!"*
- The child challenged has a choice, and answer:
  - *"Walk the Plank"*: where they will attempt to get to the ship without being tagged, or
  - *"Join the Crew"*: to give in and join the pirates.

- If the challenged child makes it safely across, they shout "Ship Ahoy", the signal for the rest to dash for safety.
- If the challenged child is caught, they join the pirate crew, while the rest of the Sailors make a dash for safety.
- Sailors making this dash may still be caught by the pirate.
- Play now resumes from the opposite end.
- At the start of the game, when there is only one or two Pegged Legged Pirates, children may only walk quickly across. Once there is three or more, children may run across.
- Play ends when all but one of the Sailors are caught. This person may become the next Pegged Legged Pirate.

7. Leprechaun Switcheroo

Equipment: One bean bag per child to mark positions

Skills: Spatial awareness, gross motor, concentration, agility

Imagery: Leprechauns are mischievous creatures who love to play tricks. Even at Leprechaun school, the little Leprechauns play tricks on their Teacher. When the Teacher is not looking, little Leprechauns catch each other's eye, wink and switch places. Ahhh, but the Teacher also knows how to play tricks on them.

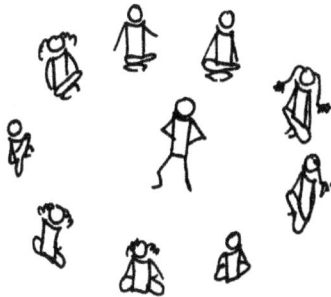

To play:
- Children are little Leprechauns sitting in a circle facing in. Bean bags are used to mark their sitting positions. One child is the Teacher Leprechaun standing in the centre.
- Children catch each other's eyes, nod or wink in agreement and switch places. When they vacate their spots, the Teacher Leprechaun tries to get to one of them.
- The Leprechaun without a seat becomes the new Teacher.
- This can get a little chaotic when more than one pair of children are attempting to swap seats. They may end up in a different vacated spot, if the Leprechaun in the middle takes their spot.

8. Toilet Flush

Equipment: Two or three red sashes, one or two blue sashes

Skills: Gross motor, agility, spatial awareness

Imagery: There is a mischievous Gremlin afoot who is causing all the toilet flushes in the land to malfunction. The toilets in the land are fearful and the plumbers are scrambling around trying to fix the problem.

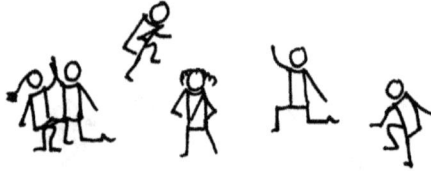

To play:
- Two or three children are Gremlins (red sash), and one or two Plumbers (blue sash). All others are Toilets fearful of malfunctioning.
- Gremlins chase after Toilets. A tagged Toilet goes down on one bended knee, and puts up the opposite hand, bent at the elbow (like a flush).
- Plumbers have to spot malfunctioning Toilets and repair them by sitting on their knee and flushing them (by gently straightening the bent arms and bringing them down).
- The game goes on endlessly until the Teacher calls for a change of Gremlins and Plumbers.

9. Cat and Mouse (3)[57]

Equipment: None

Skills: Spatial awareness, agility, quick reaction

Imagery: Cat and Mouse were once very good friends, but they had a falling out. The Cat accuses the Mouse of being cunning and the Mouse accuses the Cat of being lazy. And now whenever they meet, tensions flare! (For the story, see Cat and Mouse (1)).

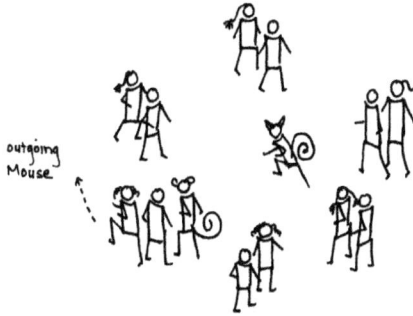

To play:
- One child is Cat and another is Mouse. All others are standing in pairs, one in front of the other. They are mice in a safe house which has only room for two mice.
- The Cat chases the Mouse, who finds safety by standing in front of a pair. This releases the child at the rear who becomes the new Mouse.

---

[57]   In this version, children form safe houses, standing in pairs, one in front of the other, giving protection to the Mouse. This is spatially more demanding as there is movement in all directions, but mostly danger comes from what is front of them.

- When the Cat catches the Mouse, they swap roles immediately.
- The game continues, until everyone has had a go.

Variation:
- Cats and Mice in Pairs: Pairs of Cats chase pairs of Mice, played as above.

10. Fox and Geese

Equipment: A soft dodge ball

Skills: Spatial awareness, agility, teamwork, ball handling skills

Imagery: Mr Fox has found his way into the goose-shed and is trying to tag a gosling for lunch. Mother Goose is very protective and does her best to fend off hungry Mr Fox!

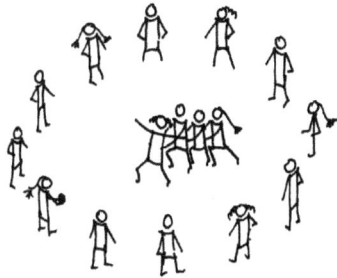

To play:
- Divide the children into groups of four, each group remembering who their teammates are.
- Set up a large circle as the goose-shed, with the first group of four standing within. One of the four is Mother Goose, and the others are Goslings standing behind her, each holding on to the waist of the person in front.
- All other children stand around but may not enter the goose-shed. One child has a ball (the Fox) and begins by trying to aim the ball at the Gosling at the rear of the line (from the knees down).
- If Little Gosling has been tagged, the tagger's team swaps places with the team in the circle.
- Tagger becomes Mother Goose, unless they have had a turn previously. Allow team members to take turns at being Mother Goose if they so desire.

11. Budge

Equipment: Two or more sashes, gym mats, rubber discs, benches

Skills: Spatial awareness, gross motor, agility

Imagery: The space around you is the ocean. There has been a ship-wreck, and bits of driftwood are bobbing around. Some sailors are clinging to these bits of driftwood and some are swimming in the water. And then they spy sharks swimming towards them. What are they going to do?

To Play:
- Set up the play area with driftwood (e.g. gym mats, rubber discs, benches) scattered around. These are safe spots, but there is only enough space for about half of the Sailors. Specify how many may be on each of these safe spots.
- Choose two or more Sharks (identified with coloured sashes) and the rest are Sailors.
- The Sharks chase the Sailors who find refuge on the bits of driftwood. Each piece of driftwood can only take a certain number of Sailors and they are only safe until a desperate Sailor budges them off.
- A budged Sailor may not go back to the same driftwood but has to swim (run) to another driftwood to budge someone else off. Sailors on driftwood are safe from shark attack.
- A Sailor who is tagged by the Shark goes to the Shark's lunch box, which has only space for three Sailors. When the fourth Sailor is squeezed into the lunchbox, the first Sailor is released.
- The game may go on endlessly until the Teacher calls for a change of Sharks, or until a Shark has caught a certain number of Sailors.

12. Paper, Scissors, Rock (1)[58]

Equipment: None

Skills: Skill, agility, quick reaction, teamwork, listening

Imagery: There were once three warriors from three kingdoms. Each was unbeaten in their own land, for there was none equal to them in strength, flexibility or precision. The Paper was the origami master and could fold around and wrap anything in its path. The Scissors ruled over the fabric kingdom for it was sharp and precise. The Rock could pound anything standing in its path.

One day, the three warriors decided to travel out in search of a worthy opponent. They met by chance one day, and there, Rock found itself wrapped up beautifully by Paper, Paper found itself cut by Scissors and Scissors found itself pounded by Rock. They were thrilled to have finally met their match that they became firm and fast friends, but they do enjoy a little rivalry every now and then.

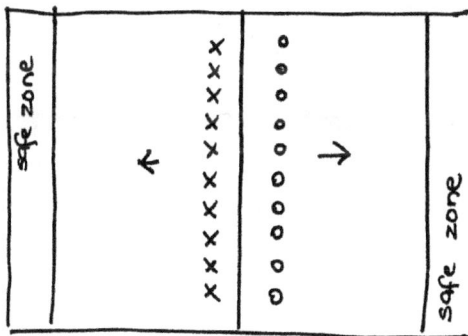

---

[58] Reputed to be the oldest hand game ever played. It is called by various names: Rock Paper Scissors, Scissors Paper Stone, Scissors Paper Rock or Roshambo.

To play:
- Establish two boundary lines at opposite ends of the play area as the safe zone, and a centre line dividing the area into two zones.
- Divide the class into two groups. Each group huddles up and chooses a group response: Paper, Scissors or Rock.
- The actions are: 'Paper': hold hand out flat; 'Scissors': extend index and middle fingers; 'Rock': - show fist.
- Their relative strengths: Paper beats Rock, Rock beats Scissors and Scissors beats Paper.
- The teams come to the centre line, standing face to face, a few paces apart. Children have one hand held in a fist in front of them.
- At a signal from the Teacher, each group counts down with a chant "Paper, Scissors, Rock". At the word "Rock", players show their response.
- The group with the stronger response chases the other group. Tagged players joins their taggers.
- The game ends when all players are on one group, or after a certain number or children are caught.

Variations:
Jump three times, and on the third jump, land in position: Paper (legs apart, arms wide), Scissors (legs in lunge, arms clasped overhead), Rock (legs together, arms crossed at chest).
- Instead of a group response, children make their own responses. The stronger response chases the weaker, and the tagged join their taggers. Play continues till all players are on one team, or after a certain number of players are left in a team.

13. Hunters, Hares and Hounds (3)[59]

Equipment: A soft dodge ball

Skills: Gross motor, ball handling skills, spatial awareness

Imagery: It's early in the morning and hunters have gathered to go hare hunting. Because of the dense cover and gnarly tangles of briar, thorns and honeysuckle, they have brought their trusty Hound to trail after the hares. All are dreaming of Stewed Hare at the end of the day.

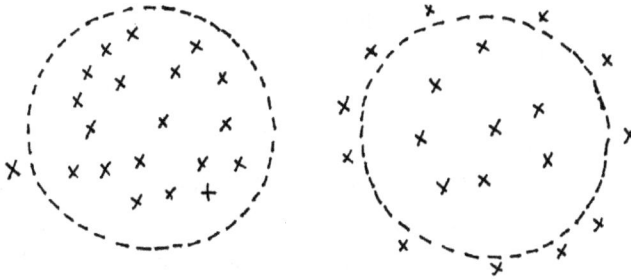

To play:
- Set up an area with rope or cones that is large enough for the whole class to run and dodge.
- All children are Hares standing in the middle, except one child (Hunter) who stands outside this area. The Hunter has a Hound (ball).
- The Hunter aims to tag a Hare (knees down). A tagged Hare joins the Hunting team with no replacement.
- The game ends when all the Hares have been caught.

Variation:
- Add an extra ball.

---

[59]   This version: circle formation, underarm toss with no replacement – tagged child joins taggers to get all hares out.

14. Giants, Wizards and Dwarfs[60]

Equipment: None

Skills: Skill, strategy, agility, spatial awareness

Imagery: The Giants who live high up in the mountains have enormous strength and a roar like thunder. They carry huge clubs, and this terrifies all the villages around the mountains. The Dwarfs live deep beneath the earth, and busy themselves mining gemstones. They may be small, but they are cunning and carry magic blades with handles encrusted with gems. The Wizards live deep in the forests practicing their magic, and dislike being disturbed.

The Giants, Wizards and Dwarfs do not usually stray far from their territory, but one day, they encountered each other! The Giants roared and clubbed the Dwarfs with a single blow but were no match for the Wizards' magic. The Wizards however, overlooked the size of the Dwarfs and their cunning ability to sneak up from below to stun them with their magic blade.

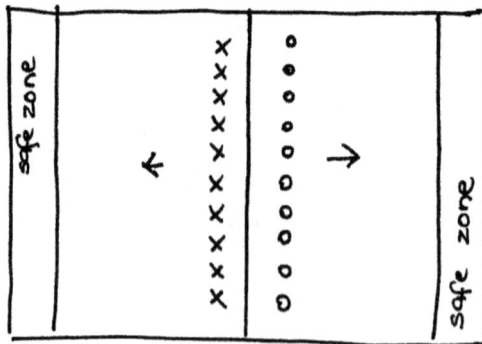

---

[60]   This is another game that revolves around the Paper, Scissors, Rock relationship.

To Play:
- Establish two boundary lines at opposite ends of the play area as the safe zone, and a midway line dividing the area into two zones.
- Divide the class into two groups. Each group huddles up and chooses a group response – Giants, Wizards or Dwarfs.
- The actions are: Giants – raise one hand as if holding a club and roar "Urrrgggghhh"; Wizards - hold both hands out in front at chest level and go "Zzzzzzzzzz" as if casting a spell, and Dwarfs - put their thumbs up (magic blades), moving them from side to side, going "Hehehehe".
- The groups come to the centre line, standing face to face, a few paces apart. On a count of three, each group shows their group response.
- Giants beat Dwarfs, Dwarfs beat Wizards and Wizards beat Giants. The group with the stronger response chases the other group. Tagged players join their tagger's group.
- Repeat until all players are on one side, or at the Teacher's discretion.

Variations:
- Dragon, Knight and Princess: The Dragon is stronger than the Princess, who is stronger than the Knight, who is stronger than the Dragon. The Dragon roars as if breathing out fire; the Princess stands tall and proud, with her hands on her head as if holding her crown, while the Knight flashes his sword.

15. Your Majesty, May I?

Equipment: None

Skills: Gross motor, spatial awareness, listening, attention, agility

Imagery: The King (or Queen) of the Land of Manners is very particular about good behaviour and manners. He loves it when his ministers and subjects say "Please", "Thank You", "May I" and "You're Welcome". And he also loves it when they listen to instructions and follow his orders. As a King, he sometimes has to give important instructions that are difficult to explain, but need to be obeyed. So the King plays this game with his Ministers, to teach them good manners and listening skills.

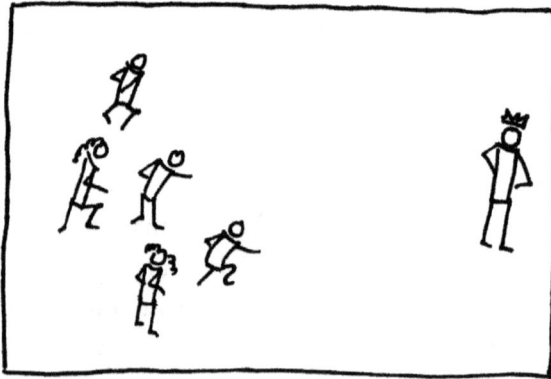

To play:
- Designate a King or Queen (usually the Teacher or have two or more Majesties) and all others are Ministers of the Court.
- The King stands at one end of the play area, with his back to the children standing at the other end.

- Ministers take turns asking, "Your Majesty, may I _____" (make a movement forward in any manner, such as "take three giant steps forwards").
- The King replies with "Yes, you may" or "No you may not, but you may____" for example ".....take two giant steps forwards instead" or "......skip five steps backwards instead".
- The King may also place conditions: "If you are wearing red, you may take three giant steps forwards".
- Ministers always obey The King's instructions.
- The game ends when the first Minister reaches The King, and this Minister becomes the new King.

Variations:
- Use 'Your Highness' and 'Subjects' or 'Captain' and 'Crew' or 'Mother' and 'Children' and tweak the story line.
- Suggestions for movements can include: Frog hops, bunny hops, crab crawl, jumping jacks, bear walk, scissor steps. Be creative and imaginative.

16. Fruit Salad

Equipment: One bean bag per child to mark sitting positions

Skills: Gross motor, attention, listening, quick reaction

Imagery: The fruits in the fruit basket are watching anxiously as the Salad Maker decides which fruit should go into the Fruit Salad for morning tea. When the Salad Maker calls out the name of a fruit, they race to see who will be safe from being cut up!

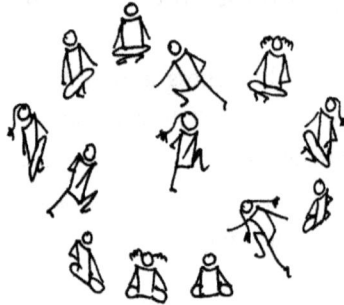

To play:
- The children sit in a circle facing inwards (use bean bag to mark their spots) while the Salad Maker, stands in the middle.
- Choose five fruits or more, and going around the circle, assign each child the name of a fruit, repeating the sequence till all have been named.
- The Salad Maker calls out the name of a fruit and those called quickly get up to change places. The Salad Maker meanwhile, slips into one of the newly vacated spots and the child without a seat becomes the new Salad Maker.
- At "Fruit Salad", all must swap places, but not with the person immediately to their left or right.

Variations:
- All children are animals at the Zoo and are assigned the name of an animal. The Zoo Keeper is taking the morning roll call, and whichever animal he calls have to swap seats. When he calls "Animal Farm", all animals to swap seats.
- Line formation is an option for older children ready for some competitiveness (Class 4). They sit in lines of five or more, with each assigned the name of a fruit or animal. One child is the caller (Salad Maker or Zoo Keeper) who stands in the front facing the others. Whichever fruit or animal is called, those so assigned have to race to the front of the line going around the first child, then race to the back around the last child in line and return to their seats. The last to return swaps places with the caller.

17. Goblins' Whispers[61]

Equipment: None

Skills: Attentive listening, visual / auditory memory, eye-hand coordination, communication skills

Imagery: A gaggle of Goblins one day, decided that they have had enough of stinging nettle soup and wanted a proper feast of wild rabbit! So they went a hunting. When the first goblin spotted a rabbit, he whispered to the next goblin to pass a message: "Send reinforcements, we are going to advance". However, reinforcements never came. Instead, there was a great cheer from the rear, when they received the message: "Send three or four pence, we are going to a dance!"[62]. Needless to say, there was no stewed rabbit and no dance that day.

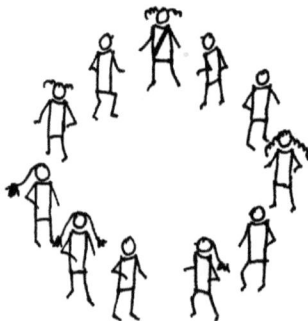

To play: • Ideal size of between 5 – 20.
• The children stand in the circle. One child is chosen to start by whispering a message to the two children on either side of him, while all others look or turn away.

___

[61]   Also knowns as Chinese Whispers, or Broken Telephone, the origins are unclear. Its entertainment value comes in comparing the original and the final message.

[62]   From the annuals of British military folklore of World War I (Rooney, 2011).

- The two children then tap the shoulders of the person next in line and whisper the message they heard. This continues, with each child in turn passing on what they think they heard, until it reaches the end person in their line (or half of the circle).
- The two last children then say aloud what they heard and compare how it has morphed from the original message.

Variations:
- Instead of a whispered message, play Telephone Charade. The starting child makes a simple gesture or action, shown only to the two children on either side, and they in turn relay that to the person next to them.

18. Saint George and the Dragon

Equipment: None

Skills: Spatial awareness, agility, quick reaction

Imagery: At the foot of Dragon Mount, a fire breathing dragon has woken from its slumber and is terrorising the villagers. Into the village rides Saint George, and the people implore him to save them from a fiery death.

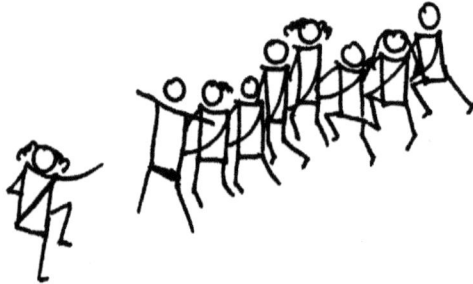

To play:
- One child is Saint George and one child is the Dragon's Head, and another is the Dragon's Tail. All others stand in a line between the Dragon's Head and Tail, each holding on to the waist of the person in front.
- Saint George's task is to tag the Tail, which is the weakest part of the Dragon. When tagged, the Tail becomes the new Saint George, Saint George becomes the new Dragon Head, and the Dragon Head moves down the line, to stand behind the new Dragon Head.
- The game ends when all players have had a chance to become Saint George, Dragon's Head or Dragon's Tail.

Variations:
- The Dragon's Head can bite! If Saint George is tagged by the Dragon's Head, they are out, and they cycle through the players as above, Saint George to Dragon's Head, Dragon's Head moves down the dragon line and the Tail becomes the new Saint George.
- For older children (Year 4 onwards), when Saint George tags a Tail, the Tail sits out in Heaven to await rebirth. When the fourth tagged Tail arrives in Heaven, the first tagged Tail re-joins the game as the Dragon's Head. When Saint George is bitten (tagged) by the Dragon's Head, he too goes to Heaven and wait in line, and is replaced by the Tail in play.

Year Four: (Ages 9 - 10)

Developmental Picture of the Ten-Year-Old:

Polarity

This is the 'heart of childhood'. The child is more 'awake' and aware of their surrounding space (both literally and inwardly). Physically, they are more capable, energetic and have more stamina. They show an increasing awareness of their own individuality, a determination and inner authority that is based on their developing moral strength, courage and responsibility.

Their ability to think and reason increases. The child begins to see that the world has flaws and is ready to question and challenge authority, yet their imaginative capability is still strong. Learning and respecting rules involved in games can help them develop their social and moral compass[63].

The child experiences polarities – dreaming and awakening, weak and strong, safety and danger, creation and destruction – the rhythm of breathing, of expansion and contraction. The child feels strongly but does not know what to do with these feelings. They struggle with their individuality and peer pressure and experience isolation from the group.

---

[63] (Rawson, 2008)

Movement Emphasis for Year 4

- Games still have an imaginative element, and focus on physical orientation, dexterity, listening, and attentiveness.
- The spaces above/below, right/left, forwards/backwards and their integration are worked on.
- Rough and tumble play comes in this year, allowing children to explore initiative, bravery, courage, reflection and agility, chasing and catching, and teach social responsibility and moral awareness. They provide an outer expression to the inner changes that children are experiencing.
- Games now involve a more rapid exchange of roles (from chaser to chased); having a specific goal (e.g. fire and ice, hunters and hares); those that pit the individual against the group; games with some image of confrontation with a negative force (river bandits, shark's jaws), and those that involve throwing and catching in increasingly difficult situations[64].

The Teacher's Sheath of Authority:

Darius II

The ten-year-old sees that the world has flaws, that the world is not black and white but many shades of grey. It is the teacher's task to unite this seeming chaos into a coherent whole.

Dan Freeman[65] suggests the image of Darius II for this age group. Darius the Great (522-486 BCE) was the third Persian King of the Achaemenid Empire. He conquered the warring Persian tribes and united them into a great Persian Empire. He restored order, kept peace, practiced tolerance, brought new ideas into Persia and expanded the Empire. Thus is the role of the Year 4 teacher.

---

[64] (Rawson, 2008)

[65] Personal communication

1. Ship Shark Shore

Equipment: Cones or rope to mark boundary lines

Skills: Listening, attention and focus.

Imagery: All players are pirates, and they know they have to follow the Captain's orders as the sea can be a treacherous place. There are only three safe spots: on the Ship, on the Shore, or on the back of a Shark. Failure to follow orders quickly and correctly could see them ending up in the Shark's lunch box.

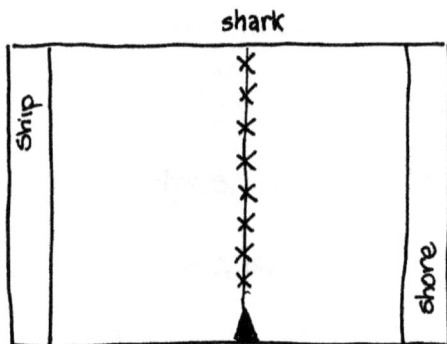

To play:
- Establish two boundary lines at opposite ends of the play area as safe zones (one is 'Ship', and the other is 'Shore') and a centre line dividing the area into two zones (the back of the 'Shark').
- All players are pirates standing straddled across the back of the Shark, and the Teacher stands at the head of this line, facing them. The Shark's lunch box is next to the Teacher.
- The Teacher barks a command (Ship, Shark or Shore) and the crew have to respond quickly and correctly by running to the correct safe zone. Those who respond incorrectly or are the slowest, will be sent to the Shark's lunchbox, which

has space for only three crew. When the fourth crew is squeezed in, the first crew pops out and re-joins the game.

- The Teacher then barks another command and the crew have to respond. The game can go on endlessly and ends at the Teacher's discretion.

2. Cut the Cake

Equipment: None

Skills: Spatial awareness, agility, quick reaction

Imagery: The Queen of Tarts loves her cakes and tarts. She however has a magic knife that likes to play tricks on her. Whenever the knife slices through the cake, it makes a cut, ah, but there is a twist! The cut is not where you think it is supposed to be.

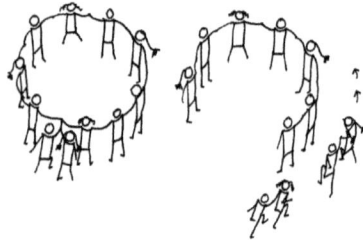

To Play:
- Two children are the Knife pair. All others are the Cake, standing in a circle, holding hands.
- The Knife pair walks around the outside of this circle, holding hands, choosing a connection between any pair of children to 'Cut the Cake'.
- They find a pair and with a gentle slicing motion, bring their arms down to break this connection.
- The two children whose connection was sliced, now reconnect, but drop the hands of the person to their other side, becoming the Cake Pair.
- Both the Knife and Cake pair quickly run in opposite direction around the circle and try to get back to the opening in the circle first.
- The first pair back to the opening becomes part of the circle while the second pair back begins the new round as the Knife and get to Cut the Cake.

3. Dragon's Treasure

Equipment: Five hula hoops, lots of bean bags

Skills: Strategy, agility, speed, cooperation

Imagery: Deep in a cave and high up in the mountains, there lives a fire breathing Dragon, who guards a horde of treasure. The villages nearby hear about the treasure and send their brave hunters to steal them. However, being greedy, they refuse to share and start to steal each other's treasures too.

To play:
- Place a hoop in the centre of the play area (the Dragon's Lair) filled with bean bags (treasures) and four hula hoops (Villages) at equal distance away from the lair.
- One child is the Dragon who guards its Lair, and all others are Villagers, divided into four equal groups, each standing behind their hula hoop,
- At the signal to start, one child from each village runs to the dragon's lair and tries to steal a treasure and bring it back to their village without being tagged by the Dragon. On returning, they place the stolen treasure into their hoop, high five the next person in line to go raiding.
- If tagged, they surrender any stolen treasure in their possession, and return home, empty handed, going to the end of the line.
- The next villager in line then sets out to steal another treasure. They may also raid each other's treasure chest.
- The game ends when one village has stolen a predetermined number of treasures.

4. Fire and Ice

Equipment: None

Skills: Teamwork, cooperation, social interaction

Imagery: In a far-away land, there lived two different peoples[66]: those who wielded the magic of fire, and those the magic of ice. They knew that one magic was not necessarily better than the other and that when they came together, their lives would be happier and they would be stronger. However, standing between them was the jealous Giant, who taunts and dares them and tries to prevent them from coming together. The Giant knew that if they were united, they would be stronger than the Giant, and would be free.

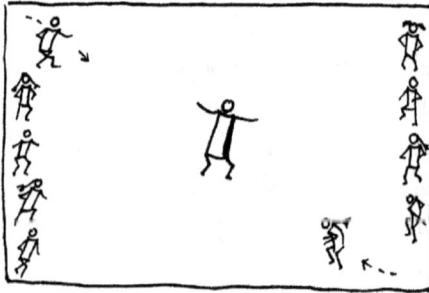

To play:
- Two equal groups, (Fire and Ice) standing in a line facing each other at opposite ends of the play area.
- One child is the Giant, who stands in the middle of the play area, and dares the others:
  Fire and Ice, come to me!
  Come to me and be free!

---

[66] This story is reproduced from (Brooking-Payne, 1998) and is used with permission.

- At this, coming from diagonally opposite directions, one person in Fire and one person in Ice come to the middle and try to touch each other, without being tagged by the Giant. If they are successful, Ice goes over to the Fire group and Fire goes over to the Ice group.
- If the Giant tags one of the pair, the tagged runner becomes the new Giant, the Giant goes to the tagged runner's group, and the other runner returns to the group they came from.
- The new Giant repeats this dare and the game goes on.
- If the Giant fails to tag anyone after three tries, a new Giant is chosen.
- The game ends after a specified time or at the Teacher's discretion.

Variation:
- Four groups: Fire, Ice, Earth and Wind, coming from four different directions, while the Giant tries to thwart their coming together.

5. Dog and Bone (or Heads and Tails)

Equipment: None

Skills: Spatial awareness, agility, cooperation

Imagery: We know how dogs love to chew on their bones and will do anything to protect their bones from other dogs. Dogs can also be greedy and will try to steal another dog's bone. So one day at a dog party, all the dogs were given a bone, but one dog decided it wasn't satisfied with just one bone!

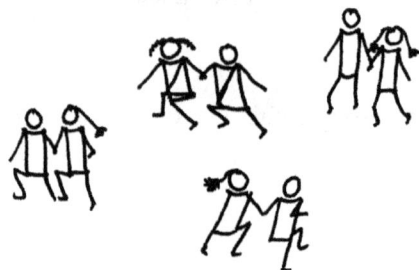

To play:
- Children stand in pairs, holding hands. The one standing on the right is a Dog, who has to protect the one standing to its left (the Bone).
- One pair is the Greedy Dog and Bone pair who tries to steal (tag) another Dog's Bone. This pair starts by giving chase.
- When a Bone has been tagged, the pair becomes the next chasing pair. They count, slowly and aloud "1, 2, 3" before giving chase.
- Pairs must remain linked at all times. If the chasing pair breaks contact, the tag is not valid. If a dodging pair breaks contact, they become the new chasers.
- Swap roles after a few rounds.

6. Captain's Orders

Equipment: A place marker for the brig

Skills: Gross motor, quick reaction, listening, focus

Imagery: All players are Crew on board a ship, sailing the treacherous seas. The Captain needs to train his men to obey his commands, as their lives may depend on how quickly they respond! Slackers will be sent to the brig (the prison)!

To play:
- Teacher is the Captain, all others are the Crew, spread out in a given area (the deck of the ship). Mark an area for the Brig.
- The Captain barks a command and the crew responds. Crew who do not follow the commands correctly or is the slowest will have to go to the Brig.
- Suggested commands: use what resonates with you and introduce a few at a time.
  - *Bow* – to the front of the ship
  - *Stern* – to the back of the ship
  - *Starboard* – to the right of the ship
  - *Port* – to the left of the ship
  - *Roll Call* –stand in one straight line from bow to stern, salute the captain and say, "Aye-aye Captain!". Remain at attention until the Captain salutes and says "At ease"
  - *Scrub the deck* – crouch down and pretend to scrub the deck
  - *Hit the deck* – lie down on their tummies
  - *Captain's wife* – curtsey
  - *Crow's Nest* – stand on one leg (mast), other foot resting on knee of standing leg (crow's nest), hands above eyes (as if scanning over the horizon)

- *Submarines* – lie on floor with one foot raised like periscope
- *Mutiny* – run around the play area sword fighting with everyone
- *Man Overboard* – sink down holding nose with hand, raising other hand in air as if going under water
- *Lifeboats* – find a partner, sit on the floor facing each other, holding hands, and rock forward and back, like rowing a boat
- *Shark Attack* - the captain becomes a shark and has 10 seconds to tag as many crew as he can. Tagged crew go to the Brig
- *Jail Break* - run to the Brig and help release their mates. Those saved can re-join the game. Give everyone a chance to get out of the Brig during Jail Break
- *Pirates* - closes one eye, puts up a hook finger, hobbles around like they have a peg leg and say "Aaargh!"

7. Cat and Mouse (4)[67]

Equipment: None

Skills: Agility, quick reaction, flexibility

Imagery: Cat and Mouse were once very good friends, but they had a falling out. The Cat accuses the Mouse of being cunning and the Mouse accuses the Cat of being lazy. And now whenever they meet, tensions flare! (For the story, see Cat and Mouse (1)).

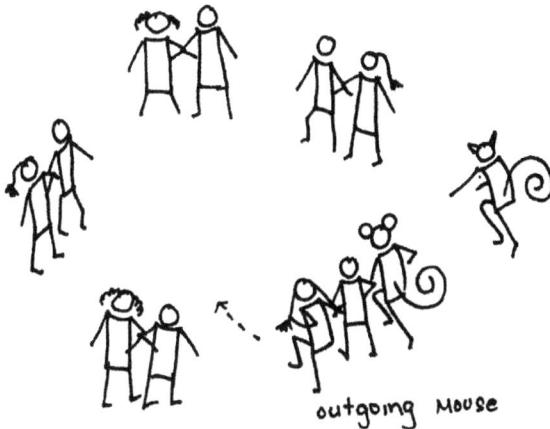

outgoing Mouse

To play:
- One child is Cat and another is Mouse. All others are pairs of mice in safe houses, standing side by side, linking arms.
- The Cat chases the Mouse, who finds a safe house by standing next to, and linking arms with one of a pair of mice. This releases an outgoing Mouse on the other side of the pair.

---

[67] In this 'side by side' version, the incoming mouse releases the mouse standing on the other side. Spatial demands increase as danger now comes from the periphery.

- The game continues, until everyone has had a chance to play. Consider bobbing down if they have had a go to ensure everyone gets a turn.

Variations: • Can be played in pairs. One pair of children is a Cat, one pair is a Mouse and two pairs of children are a safe house. An incoming Mouse pair releases the Mouse pair on the other side.

8. Hunters, Hares and Hounds (4)[68]

Equipment: One soft foam ball

Skills: Spatial awareness, agility, cooperation

Imagery: It's early in the morning and hunters have gathered to go hare hunting. Because of the dense cover and gnarly tangles of briar, thorns and honeysuckle, they have brought their trusty Hound to trail after hares. All are dreaming of stewed hare at the end of the day.

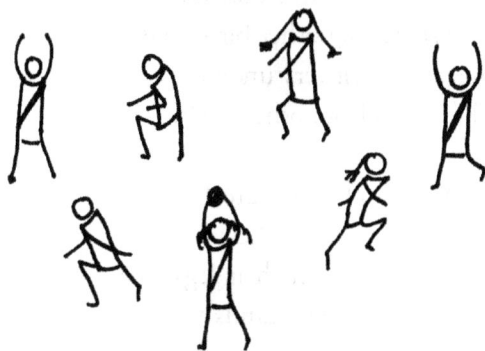

To play:
- Two students are Hunters who have a ball (Hound) between them. The rest are Hares. Hares may not touch the ball.
- Hunters tag Hares by hitting them with a dodge ball (below the shoulders). Once tagged, Hares become Hunters and join in the Hunt. Hunters may not run when in possession of the ball.
- The game ends when all the Hares have been tagged. The last two Hares may become the new Hunters.

---

[68] This version: full court with no replacement. Tagged child joins hunters till all hares have been caught.

9. Tail Tag

Equipment: One sash per child

Skills: Developing back space awareness

Imagery: Mr Peacock is very proud of his tail feather. He preens and prances around and exclaims: "Am I not the handsomest bird ever?". One day, he sees a bird with a magnificent tail and knew immediately that no other bird deserved it more than he. So he sneaks up on the unsuspecting bird and snatches its tail feather! Mr Peacock became obsessed with having more feathers so he starts snatching other birds' tails. Now the poor birds without tail feathers felt very underdressed, and they too, started to steal tail feathers from other birds.

To play:
- All the children are birds, each with a tail (sash tucked into the back of their pants), making sure that it is hanging down between their legs). They may not hold on to their tails with their hands.
- Birds start chasing each other, trying to steal another's tail while protecting their own. They may accumulate as many tails as they can, just tucking it next to their other tail(s).
- A bird with a lost tail has to bob down on the spot, waits for an unsuspecting bird to fly by, and steals its tail to re-join the chase.
- The game may go on endlessly or after a bird has accumulated a certain number of tails.

Variations:
- Birds of a Feather: Players in groups of birds (colour coordinated) each group stealing the tail feathers of other groups. The game ends when one team has lost all their tail feathers.

10. Wolves and Villagers

Equipment: Two to three sashes, two to three waist bands (if required)

Skills: Teamwork, cooperation, back space awareness, agility

Imagery: Deep in the forest, there lived a pack of wolves, and just at the edge of that forest, there is a village. The children of the village love to play and hunt in the forest, but they daren't go too deep. For when the sun goes down and the moon comes up, the wolves go "OWOOOOOO!" But every now and then, the children forget, and they venture too close. And sometimes, the wolves are hungry and they come close to the village, hoping to catch a child or two, or three, for lunch!

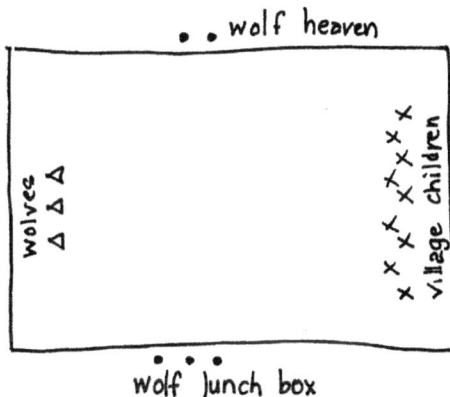

To play:
- Two or three children are the Wolves, who wear a sash as a tail (tucked into their pants or use a waist band). The rest of the children are Villagers.
- Villagers and Wolves start at opposite ends of the play area. Mark an area for the Wolves' Lunchbox and another area for Wolf Heaven.

- Children cry "Wolf King! Wolf King! You can't catch me!" To which the Wolves reply "OWOOOOO" and the chase begins.
- When children are tagged, they go to the Wolves' Lunchbox which has space for three children. But the Wolves are silly, and when a fourth child is squeezed in, the first child is pushed out, to re-join the villagers.
- The children are brave and know that if they steal a Wolf's tail, the Wolf goes to Wolf Heaven. These children then proudly wear the Wolf's tail as a trophy.
- Wolves go to Wolf Heaven and wait for re-birth – when a member of the wolf pack tags a child with the wolf tail.
- This is a game of teamwork and cooperation. The game ends when all the Wolves are in Wolf Heaven (or if the Wolves are too good and the game has gone on long enough).

Variation:
- Instead of Village children, it is the Shepherds and the Wolves.

11. Trolls (Line Tag)

Equipment: Three sashes for trolls, court with line markings

Skills: Spatial awareness, cooperation, agility

Imagery: A gaggle of trolls inhibits the mountains, and they catch unwary mountain climbers who stray into their territory, stealing their backpacks which contain troll's favourite food – granola bars!

To play:
- Three or more children are Trolls, and the rest are mountain climbers. All players begin on the lines which are mountain paths. They may not step out of line or they will fall off the mountains. They may only walk in a forward direction, or turn right or left at crossroads, but never going backwards.
- If mountain climbers meet each other, they may make room for each other to cross safely. If they encounter a Troll, they are tagged and caught, and sent hurling down the mountains, to end up in hospital. There are only enough hospital beds for four climbers, and when the fifth one is admitted, the first has to leave.
- Play goes on endlessly, until Teacher calls for a change of Trolls.

Variations:
- Trolls love stewed human beans and caught climbers end up in the troll's stewing pot. They may be saved by other climbers rescuing them one at a time. Place troll cave (mat) in a crossroad area.

12. Paper, Scissors, Rock (2)

Equipment: Cones, markers, chairs or rope, bean bags and other obstacles

Skills: Skill, strategy, agility, spatial awareness

Imagery: Story as in Paper, Scissors, Rock (1). This time, their rivalry takes place along the Path of Misadventure.

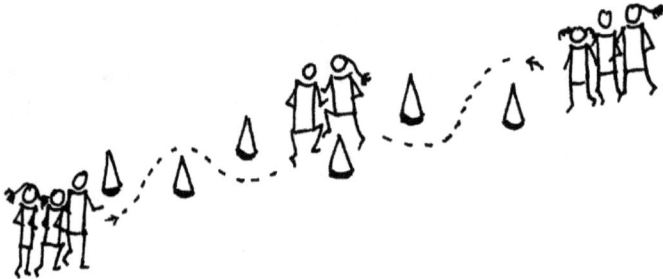

To Play:
- Divide the class into two equal groups.
- Set up a curvy line (marked by cones, markers or chairs) across the play area, with each group lining up at either end of the line, a few paces away from the last marker (that is their home base).
- At the word 'Go' the first person in the queue weaves in and out of the line in an attempt to reach the other end. When two opposing players meet, they play a game of 'Paper, Scissors, Rock'.
- The winner of that bout advances along the line as the loser drops out and returns to home base (to stand at the end of the queue for another chance).
- The retreating team immediately sends the next person in the queue to stop the other team from further advancing.

Where they meet, they play a bout of 'Paper, Scissors Rock'. One advances and the other retreats as before.

- Continue in this manner until one person in the team makes it across to the other side. This person receives a cheer, but goes back to stand at the end of their team's line to start again.
- Continue in this manner and the game can go one endlessly, until time is up.

Variations:
- Consider having two players from each team meet at a time, the second standing behind the first as a backup. If the first player is defeated and drops out, the second player quickly takes his place, while a third person quickly runs along the line to become the backup. This stops the winning team from advancing too quickly.
- For older children (Year 4) ready for some competitiveness, have a winning team. When one player makes it successfully to the other side, he waits there until all his team make it across. The game ends when one team successfully sends all their players across.
- The Path of Misadventure is full of obstacles! Place obstacles in their path, such as stations where they have to walk on tip toes, go around in spirals, tread on stepping-stones, toss some beanbags, etc.

13. Enchanted!

Equipment: Three different coloured sashes

Skills: Spatial awareness, gross motor skills, agility, cooperation, core muscle strength

Imagery: There was once a grumpy old Enchanter who did not like children. He did not like the cheery sounds of their laughter, or singing. One day, he cast several spells, turning them into rocks, trees or bridges, so he could enjoy some peace and quiet. The children are resourceful and learn to break the Enchanter's spell.

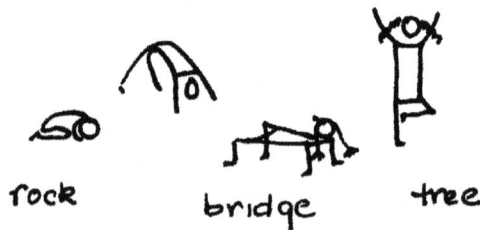

rock   bridge   tree

To Play:
- Three children are the Spells (each with a different coloured sash: e.g. Red for Rock, Blue for Bridge and Green for Tree). All others are children at play.
- Spells give chase and children dodge. Red Spell turns children into Rocks (crouch down, arms tucked); Blue Spell turns children into Bridges (in 'down dog' position: hands and feet on the ground, hip raised and head between the hands, or in 'crab' position: hands and feet on ground, hip and bottom raised off the floor); Green Spell turns children into trees (in 'tree pose' standing on one leg, with sole of

other foot resting on ankles, shin or thighs of supporting leg).

- To break the spells, free children jump over the Rocks, crawl under Bridges or run around the Trees. When freed, children may re-join the game.
- The game ends when all the children have been enchanted, or after a specified time.

14. Police and Thieves

Equipment: Six to eight hula hoops, a large quantity of bean bags, cones to mark Thieves' Hideout, basket or bucket

Skills: Spatial awareness, agility, teamwork

Imagery: A gang of Thieves break into the Museums around the country and are stealing valuable artwork. The Police chief sends in the Police force, to recover the artwork and capture the Thieves. The Thieves are cunning, and they find ways to break out of jail.

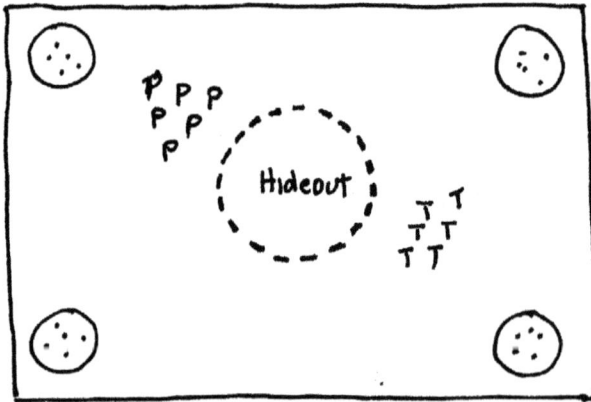

To play:
- Scatter hula hoops around the play area, and fill each with several bean bags (artwork). Set up the Thieves' hideout in the middle, with enough standing room for half the class. Place a basket to collect stolen artwork.
- Divide the class into two groups, 'Police' and the 'Thieves'. Police and Thieves begin at opposite sides of the Thieves' hideout. Thieves are safe in their Hideout.

- At the signal to start, Thieves try to steal artworks and make it safely to their hideout without being tagged. One Thief may only steal one artwork at a time.
- Tagged Thieves surrender any artwork that may be in their possession, and bob down on the spot where they are tagged. They may be rescued by a teammate who leads them back to the Hideout. They are safe as long as they are linked.
- The game ends when all art works have been stolen, or all the Thieves have been caught, or at the Teacher's discretion.
- Team swap roles after the first round.

Variation:

- Tagged Thieves go to Gaol, which is guarded. They may be saved by another Thief running to and touching the gaol post (or a designated part of the gaol boundary) without being tagged. When that happens, they shout "Gaol break" and all Thieves in the Gaol may break out. They have 5 seconds to break out and may be recaptured at any moment once they step out of Gaol.

15. The Ugly Ogres

Equipment: Two sashes, marker for Kitchen Bench

Skills: Spatial awareness, compassion, agility

Imagery: Mr and Mrs Ogre are a couple of hideous and smelly ogres who live in a castle deep in the woods. The children love to sneak into the castle grounds to forage for mushrooms. Now the Ogres love children, for they make a lovely stew, so they lie in wait. Children caught are sent to the Ogre's Kitchen Bench. But Ogres are a little dull and the children learn to outwit them.

To play:
- Two children are Ogres (identified by sashes). The rest are village children. Mark a spot for the Kitchen Bench.
- Ogres give chase. Tagged children are sent to the Kitchen Bench, which has room for three (or more) children. When the next child is place on the bench, the first one is pushed off.
- The game goes on until the Teacher calls for a change of Ogres.

Variation:
- Children can save each other by running to the Kitchen Bench, take a child by the hand and lead them home, where they may re-join the game.
- For older children: Children have magic charms (balls) that make them invisible to the Ogres. Those holding the charm need to throw it to those being chased to keep them safe.

16. Dodge Ball (1)

Equipment: One or more balls

Skills: Strategy, agility, ball handling skills

Imagery: Loki the trickster, has bewitched a ball with a laughing spell that sends anybody it touches into fits of hysterical laughter. He sends it into Giant Land and watches as they infect each other with the spell. They laugh so hard they have to sit out and wait till the spell is broken, that is, when the Giant who infected them is himself infected with the laughing spell. You know this is happening when you hear peals of thunder it the sky.

To play:
- The whole play area is neutral territory, and all players are Giants, playing against each other.
- Begin with a jump ball (or more) in the middle of the play area. The Teacher tosses the ball up and players scramble to gain control of the ball and use it to tag others from the shoulder (or waist or knees and below). Players may pivot on the spot but may not run with the ball.
- Tagged players sit out in a designated area, and may re-join the game when their tagger has been tagged out. If they do not remember who it was, just pick anyone still in the game and wait till that person is out before re-joining.
- If a player catches the enchanted ball thrown at them, the spell is reversed, and the thrower is hit with the laughing spell and has to sit out.
- The game ends when one person has tagged everyone with the laughing spell, or more usually the case, after a specified time.

17. Storm the Castle (1)[69]

Equipment: Six to ten bean bags of two different colours, cones, markers, rope or chalk to mark boundary, castle and dungeon

Skills: Spatial awareness, agility, strategy, speed, teamwork

Imagery: Two rival Kingdoms are always at war, each eyeing the other's riches and treasures. Both send in their Knights to storm the enemy castle to steal their treasure. Can they get away with it?

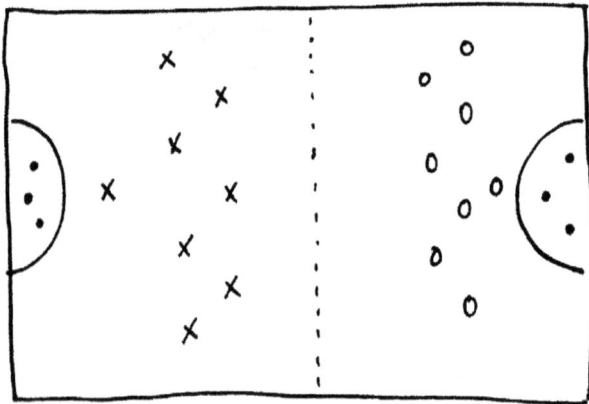

To play:
- Set up two teams and two kingdoms. Teams start in their kingdom, which is their safe zone.
- At either end of each kingdom, mark out a Castle which contains three to five beanbags (Treasures) which may be guarded by a Knight.
- At the signal to start, each invade their opponents' kingdom, to steal a Treasure, and carry it back to their Castle

---

[69] This invasion game is also known by many names, e.g. Capture the Flag, Steal the Treasure, and has many variations. In this simple version, tagged Knights simply return to their kingdom before venturing forwards again. The consequences are not as severe as in the variation where they are captured and sent to the enemy dungeon (see Storm the Castle (2), and encourages the children to participate.

without being tagged by the opponent's Knights. One Knight may only steal one Treasure at any one time.

- Knights may stay within the opponent's Castle until it is safe for them to make the dash across the centre line to their kingdom. Once they leave the Castle, they may not turn back.

- Tagged Knights must return to their Kingdom before starting out again, and any treasure in their possession when tagged has to be surrendered. The game ends when one Kingdom has stolen all the treasures.

Variation:

- Tagged Knights are sent to the Dungeon (see the Year 5 version – Storm the Castle (2)).

18. Cuckoo's Eggs (1)[70]

Equipment: Four hula hoops, four to six bean bags per team

Skills: Skill, strategy, agility, spatial awareness

Imagery: Mrs Cuckoo Bird is not your average mother bird. She is too lazy to build her own nest, instead laying her eggs in other birds' nests, leaving the tasks of raising her offspring to other birds. They can even disguise their eggs to look like the unsuspecting hosts' eggs. Well, it is Cuckoo egg laying season and Cuckoos are busy looking for nests to lay their eggs.

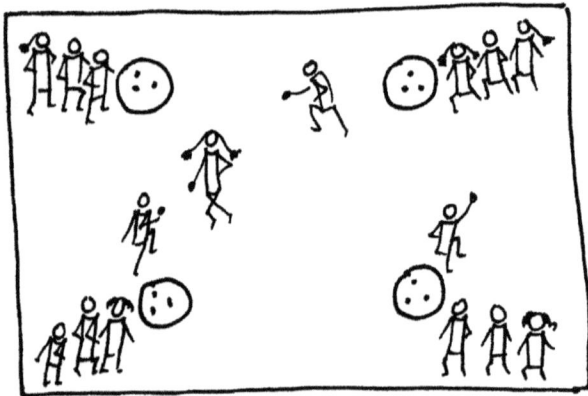

To Play:
- All children are Cuckoos. Divide the class into four equal groups, each with a Nest (hula hoop) and four Eggs (bean bags) around the play area.
- Cuckoos stand behind their Nest. At the signal to start, the first Cuckoo picks up an Egg and flies off to lay her Egg in another team's Nest. She flies back, high-fives the next bird in line, who picks up an Egg and proceeds to do the same.

---

[70] This game is a variation of Dragon's Treasure, but in reverse.

- The game ends when one group has no Eggs in their nest, or the least Eggs after a specified time.
- Birds may lay their Eggs in any Nest and have to consider other teams' Eggs in their Nest as their own and do their best to get rid of them.

Year Five: (Ages 10 - 11)
Developmental Picture of the Eleven-Year-Old:

Settled

Considered a pivotal point between childhood and puberty, between fantasy and the material world, the eleven-year-old enters a year of balance and harmony.

The child is settled, more physically coordinated, and inhabits their body in a more harmonious and integrated way. They have a sense of joy, grace, beauty and positivity about them. They are more self-assured, ready for more challenges and begin to identify their own strengths and establish their individuality. Their thinking and reasoning are more active, and they begin to think in concepts, although the pictorial aspect is still strong.

From an evolution of consciousness perspective, the 10 to 11-year-old fits into the epoch of Greece, the beginnings of democracy and the physical perfection of the Greeks and the aesthetic value of their public games. In Waldorf schools, the curriculum is imbued with the mood of the Greek Olympics, with the five major disciplines that help harness virtues such as rhythm and balance, effort and will power, focus and direction, harmony and connectedness, and centeredness.

Movement Emphasis for Class 5

- The focus is on spatial orientation, coordination, rhythm and concentration.
- Children are ready to transition from the mainly cooperative approach of group games into individual competition. Games also act as a bridge between play and sports, helping the child to transition into team based sports.
- Games imagery are now given with much more matter-of-fact pictures and the children no longer need to stand in circle. They face their teachers in rows[71].

The Teacher's Sheath of Authority:

Pericles

The authority image that Freeman[72] gives for the teacher of the eleven-year-old is Pericles (495 – 429 BCE). Pericles is a prominent and influential Greek statesman and general of Athens around the time of the Persian and Peloponnesian Wars. He is credited with the development of democracy in Athens and helped make it the political and cultural centre of ancient Greece.

The teacher does not just lay down the ground rules but is open to discussions. Negotiations can begin to occur, but it has to be understood by all. Although the teacher invites the student's input, they retain the final say.

---

[71] (Rawson, 2008)

[72] Dan Freeman (personal communication)

I. Three Lands[73]

Equipment: Three gym mats, coloured sashes for each team, identical coloured markers

Skills: Spatial awareness, agility, teamwork, quick reaction

Imagery: Once upon a time, there were three Lands, each with strengths and weaknesses. Sparta was feared for its mighty warriors, Athens, named after Athena, the goddess of wisdom and warfare, was the centre of democracy. Delphi was a sanctuary sacred to the god Apollo and home to the Oracle of Pythia. Each has something the other lacks. So who is stronger than who?

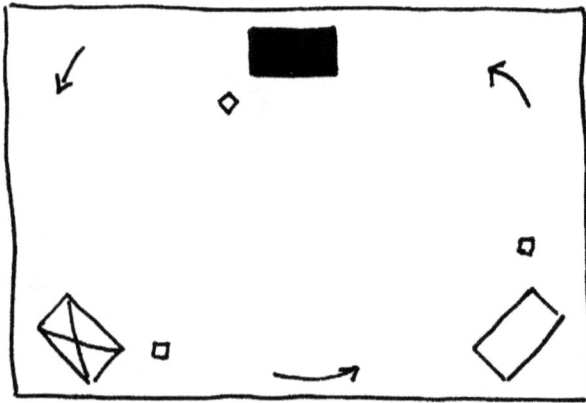

To play: • Set up three equal groups (identified by their sashes) and place three gym mats paced equilaterally apart. The distance should be far enough to run and be challenging, yet close enough to make tagging and rescuing achievable.

---

[73] A game that revolves around the Paper, Scissors, Rock relationship. I first played this game at Michael Hall Steiner School with Martin Baker, in 2009, but have since used this imagery for Year 5 that relates to their curriculum on Ancient Greece.

- Mark a spot for 'Prison', a few paces to the right of each land, in the direction of their weaker opponent. One guard may be assigned.
- Each land identifies their weaker and stronger opponents. E.g. Sparta (red) is stronger than Athens (blue), who is stronger than Delphi (yellow), who is stronger than Sparta.
- All players start off on their land, and the objective is to capture as many of their weaker opponents while evading capture by their stronger opponents.
- All players are safe only when they have both feet on their land, including those guarding the Prison.
- A tagged player goes to Prison and is rescued by a team member leading him by the hand, back to their Land. They are safe from capture when they are linked, and one team member may only rescue one prisoner at a time.
- Prisoners may form a rescue chain towards their Land, with the latest prisoner having at least one foot on the Prison marker.
- The game ends when one team is all caught out or whoever has the most prisoners after a specific time.
- After a while, swap prison markers to the other side of each land and reverse the direction of the chase.

2. Chariot Fight

Equipment: One waist band each plus one 'tail' per chariot

Skills: Spatial awareness, agility, teamwork

Imagery: We are at the Hippodrome in ancient Olympia, and all is set for the Chariot Races. The horses are ready, the Charioteers are ready, but suddenly, someone steals a horse's tail! He cannot compete without a tail, so he steals another's tail, and this sets off a tail snatching frenzy!

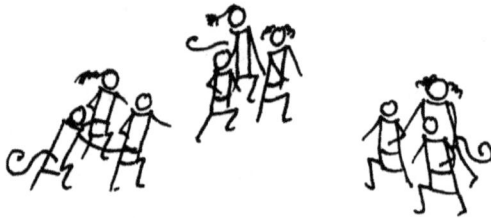

To play:
- In groups of threes, with two players (Horses), each wearing waist bands and linking their elbows. The third player (the Charioteer) stands behind the two holding on to their waist bands. The Charioteer has a tail tucked in his back.
- The Horses try to steal a Charioteer's tail while also protecting their Charioteer's tail from being stolen.
- If the charioteer loses his tail, all three bob down. They may re-join the game if one of the Horses captures the tail of a passing chariot.
- Stolen tails get tucked behind the Charioteers who stole them. Each chariot may steal as many tails as they can.
- The winner is the team with the most tails, after a specified time. Players may swap roles within their groups.

3. Noah's Ark

Equipment: None

Skills: Spatial awareness, tactics, agility, strength

Imagery: The big flood is coming, and Noah is trying to gather the animals and bring them on board the Ark. However, the animals do not understand what Noah is trying to do, so they run away from him. Noah has to show some tough love and try to catch as many animals as possible.

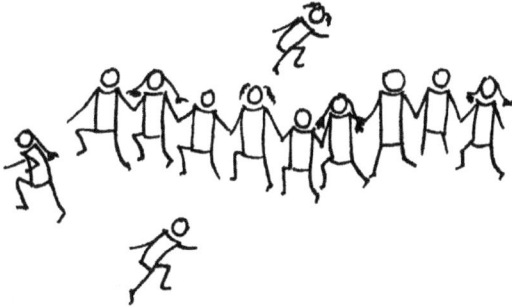

To play:
- One player is 'Noah', all others are animals.
- Noah tries to tag the animals. The first tagged animal links hands with Noah and successive animals link on to form a long chain, until all are tagged.
- The animals linked to Noah may help him chase, corner or hinder other animal's escape attempts but only Noah is allowed to tag. The link must remain unbroken to make a tag valid.
- Physical contact may be a little more robust and rough but not mean.
- The game ends when all animals are tagged.

4. Storm the Castle (2)[74]

Equipment: Six to ten bean bags of two different colours, cones, rope or chalk to mark boundary, castle and dungeon

Skills: Spatial awareness, agility, strategy, speed, teamwork

Imagery: Two rival Kingdoms are always at war, each eyeing the other's riches and treasures. Both send in their Knights to storm the enemy castle to steal their treasure. Who will be the victor?

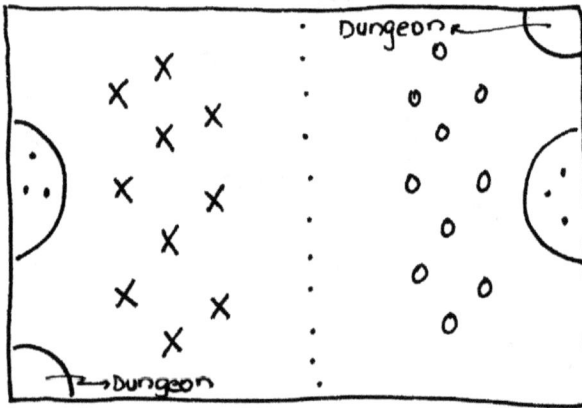

To play:
- Set up two teams and two kingdoms. Teams start in their kingdom, which is their safe zone.
- At either end of each kingdom, mark out a Castle which contains three to five beanbags (Treasures) which may be guarded by one or two Knights, and a Dungeon, which may be guarded by a Knight.
- To start, each kingdom invades their opponents' land to steal a Treasure and carry it back to their Castle without

---

74 Also known as Capture the Flag or Steal the Treasure, and has many variations. This version has a dungeon where captured enemy Knights are sent.

being tagged by opposing Knights. A Knight may only steal one Treasure at a time.

- Knights may stay within the opponent's Castle until it is safe for them to make the dash across the centre line to their kingdom. Once they leave the Castle, they may not turn back.
- Tagged Knights are sent to the Dungeon and must surrender any Treasures that may be in their possession.
- They await rescue by fellow Knights taking them by the hand and leading them across the centre line back to their kingdom. They are safe from capture when linked, and one Knight may only rescue one prisoner at a time.
- Prisoners may join hands to make a rescue chain leading towards their territory, as long as the last prisoner has at least one foot in the Dungeon.
- The game ends when one Kingdom has stolen all the treasures.

Variation:
- Limit the number of Knights allowed in the opponent's Castle at any time.
- Knights in the opponent's Castle may throw the Treasure to a fellow Knight who is also in enemy kingdom, who then has to carry it safely over the centre line to their kingdom. They may not attempt to throw it across to their own kingdom.
- Knights may not step into their own Castle but may reach in from the boundary and tag any unwary opponent Knights. If tagged, Knights have to go to the opponent's Dungeon.

5. Team Dodge

Equipment: Coloured sashes for each team, two soft dodge ball of the same colour as team sashes

Skills: Spatial awareness, agility, teamwork, ball handling skills

Imagery: Loki, the trickster has bewitched a ball with a laughing spell that sends anybody it touches into fits of hysterical laughter. He sends it into the land of the Giants and watches as tribes of Giants infect each other with the spell. They laugh so hard they have to sit out and wait till the spell is broken, that is, when the Giant who infected them is himself infected with the laughing spell. You know this is happening when you hear peals of thunder in the sky.

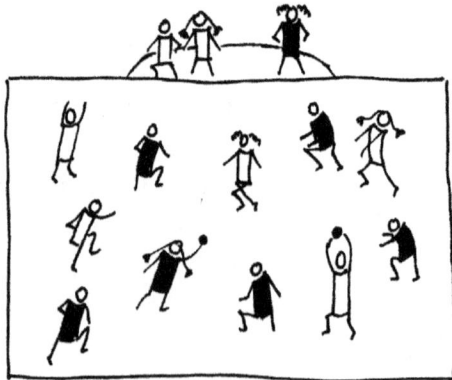

To play:
- Divide the class into two tribes, identified by sashes. One player in each tribe is given a ball and starts by aiming the ball at the opposing team (shoulders and below) to tag them out.
- Each team retains their ball and once a ball is released, only team members may collect their balls.

- Players may pivot on the spot and relay the ball to their teammates but may not run with it.
- Tagged players sit out in a designated area, and may re-join the game when their tagger has been tagged out. If they do not remember who it was, just pick someone on the opposite team still in the game and wait till that person is out before re-joining.
- If a player catches the ball thrown at them on the full, the spell is reversed and the thrower has to sit out.
- The game ends when one tribe has tagged all of the opposing tribe players (or after a specified time).

Variations:
- Balls once released, may be collected by players from either team.
- Have more balls.
- Place the balls in the middle of the play area. At a given signal, players may run to gain control of the balls.
- Have three or more tribes.

6. King Dodge

Equipment: One soft dodge ball; court with lines or chalk to draw lines, or rope /cones to mark boundaries

Skills: Spatial awareness, agility, quick reflexes, teamwork

Imagery: The invading Persian fleet has arrived on Greek soil. Outnumbered, the Athenian defenders chose their battlefield strategically: marshes on one side, mountainous terrain on the other, and lured the best enemy fighters to the centre, to meet their own. A messenger has been despatched for reinforcement. Can this small army hold on until help comes? Will it come?[75]

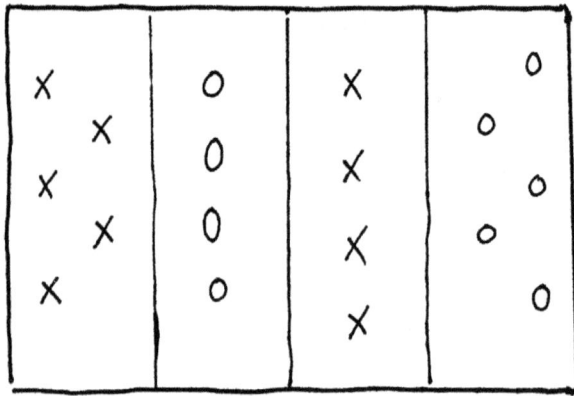

To play:
- Divide the class into two teams, Athens and Persia. Divide the play area into four zones. Zones one and four are home zones (e.g. Athens in zone one and Persia in zone four. Zones two and three are Battle zones.
- Each team begins in their home zone, where they are safe. They then send in their first group of soldiers (four to six

---

[75] Inspired by the Battle of Marathon, for which Pheidippides was said to have ran 240 km to Sparta seeking help, which never came.

depending on the size of the group and the court) into the battle zones: Athenians into zone three and Persians into zone two.

- Begin with a jump ball. Teacher stands in the middle of the court and tosses the ball into the air, and one player from each team attempts to gain control of the ball.
- The aim is for each team to get their opponents in the battle zones out by tagging them with the ball (from the waist down). They may relay the ball back and forth between their home and battle zones.
- Only players in the battle zones may be tagged.
- When a player is tagged, they retire injured to the home zone, and a replacement is sent in. Each player may only be sent into the battle zone once. Retired soldiers continue to provide support to teammates in the battle zones.
- The game ends when one army has eliminated all enemy soldiers in the battle zone.

7. River Bandits

Equipment: Four – five gym mats or carpet squares, territory markers (cones, ropes or chalk to mark)

Skills: Spatial awareness, agility, strategy, teamwork, speed

Imagery: The River Bandits have a hideaway cave near the river, where they stash all the treasure they stole from boats travelling along the river. Guards are stationed near the cave. The village children hear about this jewel cave and being curious, set out to explore. Bandits capture these nosy children, lock them up, and send them off to the Pirate King on the next boat out. The children cannot leave their friends to this fate, so they sneak into the cave to rescue them.

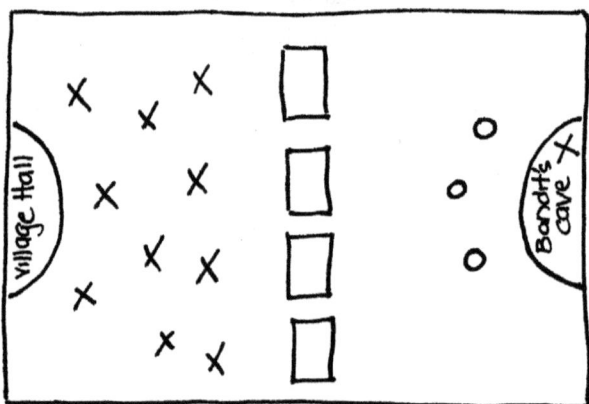

To play:
- Set up the Bandits' Cave at one end of the play area and the Village Hall at the other.
- Place gym mats at intervals in the middle of the play area to represent the crocodile infested river. The spaces in between are Bridges, the only safe way to cross.

- Three (or more) players are the Bandits; the rest are Village Children. One child has been captured and starts at the Bandit's Cave, the others in the Village Hall.
- The Bandits may roam all over the play area but may not enter the Village Hall. The Children are only safe when in the Village Hall.
- All begin in their territory. At the signal to start, children run out and attempt to save their captured teammate. To do so, they run to the cave entrance, and taking hold of their teammate's hand, lead them safely across a bridge to the Village Hall. A villager may only rescue one villager at a time, and they are safe when connected.
- The bandits try to prevent a rescue by guarding their cave and capturing the would be rescuers.
- If there is no incentive to leave the safety of the Village Hall, the Teacher may say: "Spring Cleaning" which indicates that all have to leave the Hall for it to be cleaned.
- Bandits may not 'puppy guard' the bridges.

Variations:
- Instead of only bridges, have obstacles, such as a play tunnel over a mat to indicate a Tunnel under the river and children have to crawl under to cross the river. Or a Waterfall!

8. Hunters, Hares and Hounds (5)[76]

Equipment: One or more soft dodge ball, three sashes, hula hoop or basket-ball hoop

Skills: Spatial awareness, agility, cooperation,

Imagery: Similar to Hunters, Hares and Hounds (4). This time tagged Hares go to the Picnic Basket and wait for rescue. The Hares are cheeky and clever, and they trick the Hound down a burrow where it gets stuck!

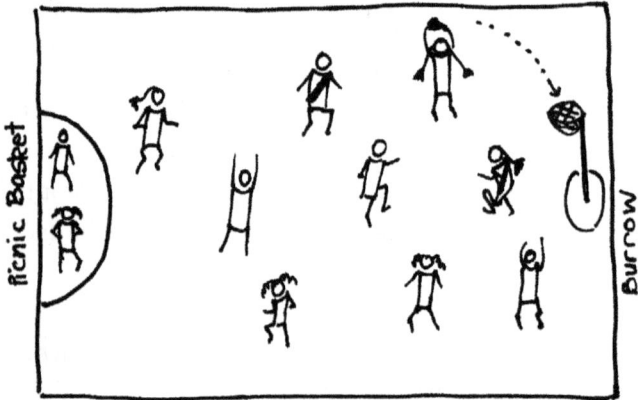

To play:
- Three students are Hunters who have a ball or two (the Hound) between them. The rest are Hares. Mark a spot for the Picnic Basket, and a Burrow (basketball hoop, hula hoop or bench).
- Hunters tag Hares (shoulders and below) and Hares dodge or intercept the ball (using forearms and hands to deflect and catch the ball). They may not run when in possession of a ball.

---

[76] This version: tagged hares go into the picnic basket and hounds may be tricked down a burrow.

- Tagged Hares go to the Picnic Basket. They are rescued and re-join the game when a Hound is tricked down a burrow and gets stuck. This could be any obstacle such a Hare scoring a ball through a basketball hoop or a Hare on a bench or in a hula hoop catching a ball thrown to them.
- The game ends when all Hares are in the Picnic Basket or after a specified time.

9. Bombardment

Equipment: Four soft dodge balls, chalk, ropes or cones to mark zones, small cones for treasures

Skills: Spatial awareness, agility, teamwork, strategy

Imagery: In a far-away land, there lived two tribes of warriors, each standing guard over three objects sacred to their tribe: a Mirror of Wisdom, a Sword of Valour and a Jewel of Benevolence. If those items were destroyed, the tribe would become weak and have to swear allegiance to the conquering tribe. Each tribe guarded their treasures for many centuries but one day, they waged war against each other, using fireballs, aiming to destroy the opponents' sacred objects.

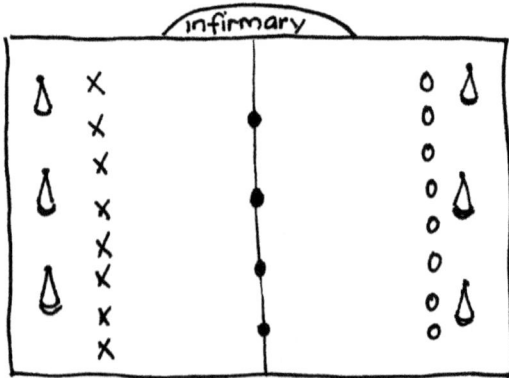

To play:
- Set up two teams and two zones. At the end of each zone, place three small cones (the treasures). Place four balls (Fireballs) on the centre line.
- Each team starts at the back of their zone. At the signal to start, teams may rush to gain control of the balls.

- The aim is to knock all the opponents' cones over and tag any opponents (below the waist) that stand in the way. It is not in the spirit of the game for players to sit, kneel or lie in front of their cones.
- Players may deflect the ball (forearms – from elbow to hands) or catch the ball on the full.
- Tagged players go to their Infirmary.
- A teammate who catches a ball on the full, may save a wounded teammate who gets to re-join the battle. The first to be wounded is the first to be saved.
- If a Fireball is caught on the full, the magic is reversed and the thrower has to go to their Infirmary, to await healing.
- The game ends when one tribe has knocked all their opponent's cones over, or all the opponents are in the Infirmary.

Variations:
- When an opponent's cone is knocked over, all the wounded players of the thrower's team are healed and able re-join the battle.
- Teacher may call "Magic Healing" and all the wounded may re-join the game.

10. Bench Ball

Equipment: Sashes for one team, one dodge ball, two benches

Skills: Throwing, catching, strategy, agility, teamwork

Imagery: Two Lords and their Knights are competing for the honour of being their King's / Queen's Elite Guards. They have to prove their worthiness at skill, agility, teamwork, stamina and chivalry by making sure that every Knight in their team gets to go on the Bench of Valour.

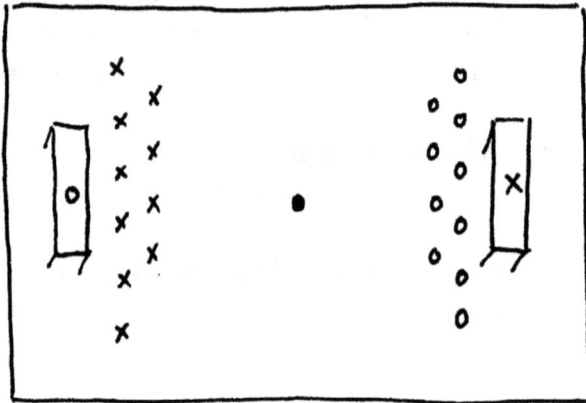

To play:
- Set up two teams (one team with sashes), and two benches at opposite ends of the play area. Each bench has to be sturdy and long enough to fit a team of players.
- The whole court is neutral territory except for the team benches.
- Each team chooses a Champion, who starts on a bench. The rest of the team start at the opposite end of the court facing their champion.

- Place a dodgeball in the centre of the court. At the signal to start, Knights from each team may rush to get control of the ball.
- Knights must relay the ball to their teammates, without it being caught or intercepted, in an attempt to pass the ball to their Champion. Knights may pivot on the spot but not run with the ball.
- When the Champion catches the ball, the thrower joins the Champion on the bench. Control of the ball then passes to the opposite team.
- As play progresses there will be more Knights on each of the benches to help their Champions catch the ball.
- When a team has two Knights remaining on the court, the Champion gets off the bench. It is the Champions' duty to help their remaining Knights get on the Bench.
- The game ends when one team has all the Knights, except their Champion, on the Bench.

Variations:
- Players must pass the ball at least three times, between teammates before throwing it to their teammates on the bench.
- If the Champion catches a ball, the thrower becomes the new Champion, and they swap places. The idea is for everyone to have a chance at being the Champion. The game ends when all players on one team has had a chance at being the Champion on the bench.

11. Cat and Mouse (5)[77]

Equipment: None

Skills: Spatial awareness, agility, quick reaction

Imagery: Cat and Mouse were once very good friends, but they had a falling out. The Cat accuses the Mouse of being cunning and the Mouse accuses the Cat of being lazy. And now whenever they meet, tensions flare! (For the story, see Cat and Mouse (1)).

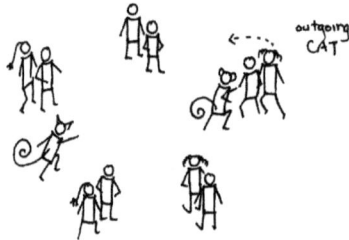

To play:
- One child is the Cat, another is the Mouse. All others standing in pairs, one in front of the other.
- The Cat chases the Mouse. If the Cat catches the Mouse, they swap roles immediately. The Mouse has to find a safe house by standing in front of a pair, to release the child at the rear, but unlike previous versions, this time, a CAT is released, and the chase begins anew.
- The game continues, until everyone has had a chance to be either the Mouse or Cat.

Variations:
- Children standing in pairs side by side. When a chased Mouse stands next to a pair, the child on the other side is released as the Cat.
- Can be played in pairs of Cats and Mice.

---

[77] This version has an added element of surprise and change as the incoming Mouse releases a Cat instead.

12. Cat and Mouse (6)[78]

Equipment: None

Skills: Spatial awareness, agility, quick reflexes

Imagery: Cat and Mouse were once very good friends, but they had a falling out. The Cat accuses the Mouse of being cunning and the Mouse accuses the Cat of being lazy. And now, whenever they meet, tensions flare! (For the story, see Cat and Mouse (1)).

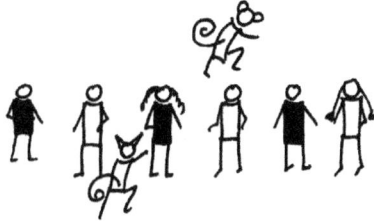

To play:
- Divide the class into two groups, one is Cat and the other, Mice.
- In the centre of the playing area, all the Cats stand in a straight line, shoulder to shoulder, with a small gap in between each, enough for a person to pass through. They alternately face in and out. One Cat is nominated to start the chase, and it stands at the start of this line.
- The Mice stand in a line parallel to and facing the Cat line, just outside the immediate play area. They nominate the first three or four Mice to enter the play area.
- At a signal, the nominated Cat begins the chase. Mice may weave in and out and run in a clockwise or anti clockwise direction around this Cat line to evade capture.

---

[78] This version sees all the cats in a line, working together to catch out all the mice.

- A Cat may only move forward, in a clockwise direction. It may not weave in and out of the Cat line but may enlist the help of a forward-facing Cat to catch Mice on the other side of the line. It does this by tapping the back of a forward-facing Cat, the signal to release it to hunt, while it steps into the vacated spot.
- A tagged Mouse is out and goes to the end of the Mice line and a new Mouse takes its place. Make sure that there is always three or four Mice in play, until there are no more Mice left to be sent in.
- The game ends when all the Mice have been caught.
- The group now swap roles, the Mice group become the Cats and the Cats become the Mice, and the process is repeated.
- The objective is for the Cats to work together to get the Mice out as fast as possible.
- A timer can be set to time each team, and the winning team is the one that catches all the mice the quickest.

13. Human Knot

Equipment: None

Skills: Teamwork, communication, problem solving, resilience

Imagery: Deep inside the labyrinth in Crete, lived the Minotaur, half man, half bull, imprisoned there by his stepfather, King Minos of Crete. He dined on human sacrifices commanded by King Minos, and supplied by the poor people of Athens, a city he had conquered. This terrible rite lasted many years. To save his people from further sacrifices, Theseus of Athens offered to enter the labyrinth and slay the monster, even though it is well known that anyone who enters is doomed to get lost and be eaten by the monster.

The King's daughter, Ariadne, fell in love with Theseus, so she gave him a ball of golden thread and told him to tie one end to the entrance and unroll the ball as he entered the labyrinth. Theseus found the Minotaur, slayed him and retraced his way back to the entrance by following the thread.

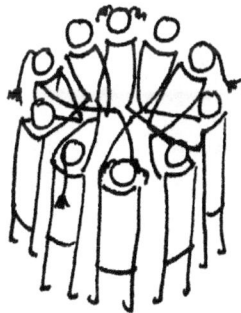

To play: •   Players form a tight circle of between six – twenty people, standing shoulder to shoulder. Reaching out first one hand

and then the other, they grasp the hands of someone in the circle, with each hand connected to a different person, thus forming a 'human knot'.

- Players attempt to unravel themselves from this knot. They may manoeuvre, bend, twist, duck under, or cross over, adjusting their grips as required, but not let go of hands.
- If the chain is broken, they have to re-start.
- General tips:
  - Try it with larger groups, the larger the group, the trickier it gets.
  - The unravelled knot may have some people facing in and out.
  - Sometimes they end up with two or more circles.
  - Sometimes the knot cannot be untangled.

14. Tic Tac Toe (Noughts and Crosses)

Equipment: For each group size of eight to ten people, you will require a 3 x 3 grid marked with nine hula hoops and twelve hoop fasteners (or marked with chalk or rope); four beanbags of one colour and four bean bags of a different colour, two starter markers

Skills: Spatial awareness, strategy, problem solving, agility, aim, core muscle strength

Imagery: Three little sailor boys went out to sea to see what they could see. Out came their telescope and high was their hope. And as they sailed, they sang and hailed: Tic tac toe, here we go, three little sailor boys in a row.[79]

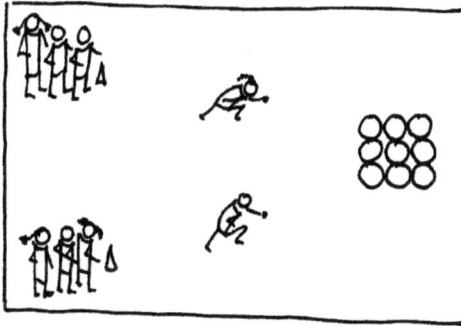

To play:
- Divide players into two groups of four to five players.
- Set up a 3 x 3 grid, and two start markers, one for each group, equidistant from the grid, at least 5 metres away (vary this for your class).
- Each group starts behind their marker. The first four in each group hold on to a bean bag of the same colour to tell them apart from the other group.

---

[79] Taking inspiration from a game of Tip Tap Toe in (Bancroft, 1909)

- At the signal to start, the first player on both teams run to toss a bean bag into a space in the grid. They return and high-five their next teammate in line to do the same. Bean bags must land within a hoop.
- Players rotate through this line until the game ends with one team having placed three bean bags in a row (vertically, horizontally or diagonally), or it ends in a draw.
- Clear the bean bags and repeat with the next person in line to re-start the game.

Variations:
- Add obstacles along the way to the grid, such as a climbing frame, crawling tunnel, jumping jacks station, etc.
- Use cones to set out a 3 x 3 grid and throw hula hoops or quoits (two different colours) around them.
- Human knots and crosses: instead of tossing beanbags, players run and stay in the grid, and they depict whether they are Noughts (sitting on the ground, curling up into a ball) or Crosses (standing with feet wide and arms out at horizontal).

15. Line Wrestle

Equipment: A straight line marked on the ground

Skills: Skill, strategy, centeredness, spatial awareness

Imagery: Gladiators often have to wrestle, especially when they have lost their shields or swords. They often have to fight to the death. The surviving Gladiator is honoured, while the rest are sent to face the lions. Who will be crowned Gladiator?

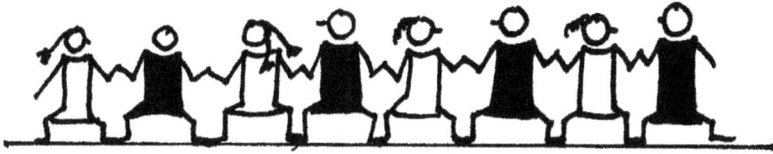

To play:
- Mark a straight line on the floor or a court with lines. Players stand on the line, almost shoulder to shoulder, with every alternate person facing the opposite direction, clasping the hands of the person next to them, and their adjacent feet touching.
- At the signal to start, players try to push or pull to unbalance others while withstanding the onslaught of the group wrestle.
- Anyone who oversteps the line, breaks their hold, or has a third point of contact with the floor (knees, hands or bottoms etc.) has to step out. The line quickly re-forms with remaining players, in whichever direction they are facing. The last person standing is crowned the champion Gladiator.

16. Line Tug of War

Equipment: Two lines marked on the ground

Skills: Skill, strength, cooperation

Imagery: In times of dispute, even before paper, scissors, rock was invented, warring parties used to settle their disputes with a game of tug of war. Here the Warlords are trying to decide who has first claims to the spoils of war.

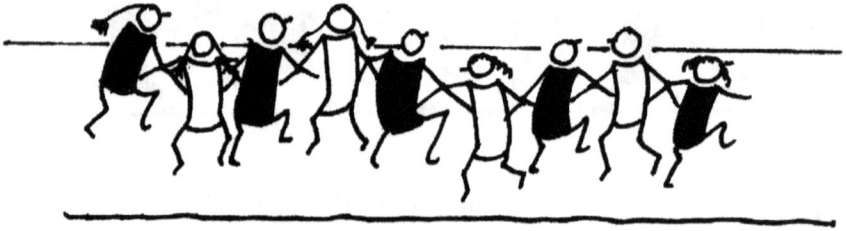

To play:
- Two boundary lines are marked on the ground, about one and a half metres apart.
- Players stand in a row, in the middle of this space, every alternate person facing the opposite direction, linking arms at the elbow.
- At the signal to start, they pull and push, each group trying to cross the line in front of them, without letting go of the link.
- The first player who makes it across the line wins the contest for their team.

Variations:
- The winning group is the one that has all its players across the boundary.

17. Four Way Wrestle

Equipment: None

Skills: Spatial awareness, agility, strategy, coordination

Imagery: Gladiators often have to wrestle with more than one opponent. The surviving Gladiator is honoured, while the rest are sent to face the lions. Who wants to face the lions?

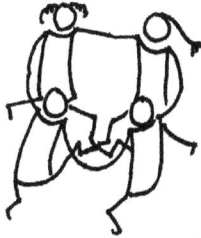

To play:
- In groups of fours, each player places one foot forward, their feet meeting at a centre point. They grasp the hands of the person next to them and prepare to wrestle.
- At the signal to start, players tug and pull to unbalance their opponents. If their opponents lift up a foot, or fall over, or have a third point of contact with the floor (e.g. hand, knee, or bottom), that player is out.
- Players quickly re-group and continue wrestling till only one player is left.

Variations:
- Groups of other sizes from three to six work well too. Eliminate till only one player is left.

18. Cuckoo's Eggs (2)[80]

Equipment: Six to eight hula hoops per team plus one for the centre, four bean bags per team

Skills: Skill, strategy, agility, spatial awareness

Imagery: It is well known that Cuckoos lay their eggs in other birds' nests and leave the tasks of raising their offspring on other birds. They can even disguise their eggs to look like the unsuspecting hosts' eggs. Well, it is Cuckoo egg laying season and Cuckoos are very busy trying to find nests for their eggs but must compete with other cuckoos doing the same.

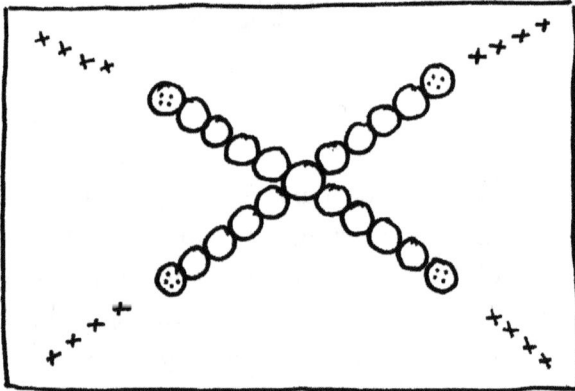

To Play:
- All children are Cuckoo birds. Divide the class into four to six equal groups, keeping group size small to reduce waiting time.
- Set up a hula hoop in the middle of the play area. For each group, place six to eight hula hoops radiating out of the centre. The last hoop of each team is their Cuckoo's Nest,

---

[80] This game is a variation of Dragon's Treasure, but in reverse, and is the advanced version of Cuckoo's Eggs, which revolves around the Paper, Scissors, Rock relationship.

containing four Eggs (bean bags). Each group starts behind their Nest.

- At the word 'Go' the first Cuckoo in each Nest picks up an Egg (bean bag) and hops with both feet together in the hoops towards any of the opposing Cuckoo's Nest to their right or left. Their objective is to drop their Egg in another group's Nest.
- When two opposing Cuckoos come head to head, they play a game of 'Paper Scissors, Rock' to determine who advances and who drops out.
- The winner proceeds while the loser returns to their nest with their Egg and goes to the back of their line and await their next turn. The losing side does not wait for their player to return but should quickly send out their next player to stop the opposing team's advancement.
- Once a player deposits an egg in an opponent's hoop, they return to their team, going to the back of the queue, while the next Cuckoo bird immediately takes off with an egg towards an opponent's nest.
- The game ends when one group has deposited all their eggs into another Cuckoo's Nest or has the least number of Eggs after a specified time.

Variation:
- Cuckoos may lay their eggs in any Nests, to the right, left or across.

Year Six (Ages 11 - 12)

Developmental Picture of the Twelve-Year-Old:

Changeling

Considered a changeling time, the twelve-year-old child is moving out of childhood into adolescence. For them, it feels like standing on the edge, in no man's land, neither truly belonging in childhood, nor in the adult world.

This is a period of considerable physical growth spurts. The child's movements become more awkward but forceful, as if they are falling into gravity. Their shoulders begin to slump with the weight of this heaviness, and they may be a little gangly, awkward and self-conscious. This is a year to strive towards uprightness and balance, and games move toward more order and structure, helping them transition to competitive team sports.

These physical changes are accompanied by an increase in cognitive ability, the capacity to understand cause and effect, and the ability to see things from another's perspective. There is a strengthening of the forces of feeling and willing, seen in their readiness to challenge the 'authority' (inner strength) of adults in their life. They have a stronger connection to and thirst for knowledge of the wider world, and an appreciation for order and structure.

Though intellectually more capable, they are still not in a position to direct these forces out of their own inner strength. They begin to take more responsibility for their behaviour, and their social relationships are characterised by strong friendships in small groups.

Movement Emphasis for Year 6

- Games and movement need to counter the fall into gravity, the heaviness of this age group, by strengthening their uprightness – which requires an inner balance of forces.
- The focus is on spatial awareness, physical activity, strength, power, speed, skills, further development of fine motor adjustments and coordination of muscular action with sense judgements, displayed individually, and also cooperatively.
- Games begin to incorporate more formal rules and arrangements and act as a transition to team sports. This age group is ready to have winners and losers, to outwit their opponents, sometimes with physical contact and to keep scores (e.g. in dodge ball, bench ball, prisoner, invasion and territorial games).[81]

The Teacher's Sheath of Authority:

Caesar

The teacher is the Caesar, the absolute law! The authority image[82] is that of Augustus Caesar (27 BCE – 14 CE) who is credited with being the greatest Roman Emperor. His official last words were, "I found Rome a city of clay but left it a city of marble" [83]which appears to reflect his achievements during his reign as emperor. He is credited with initiating two centuries of peace (the Pax Romana), and the economy, arts and agriculture flourished.

He also passed many reforms and laws, such as making adultery illegal. He strictly adhered to the laws himself, so much so that he banished his daughter and granddaughter for adultery.

---

[81] (Rawson, 2008)
[82] Dan Freeman (personal communication)
[83] (Mark, 2018)

With the child's capacity to understand cause and effect, comes a challenge for the teacher. The teacher sets the law, acknowledges if a law is broken and follows through with a consequence. A simple apology is not good enough, but rather to be followed through with an action, i.e. what needs to be done in order to make things safer, or better. By the same token, task achievements and positive behaviour are acknowledged, celebrated and rewarded.

What sets this year apart is that, for the first time, the teacher is also subjected to the same law. They are after all, Caesar!

1. Five Lands

Equipment: Five gym mats, sashes for each team, corresponding coloured markers

Skills: Spatial awareness, teamwork, agility, speed, strategy

Imagery: Five kingdoms[84] have an uneasy truce, waiting for a time to expand their territory. Each kingdom has an eye on the lands of their weaker neighbour and one day, they attack! But it seems their enemy's enemy can be their friend!

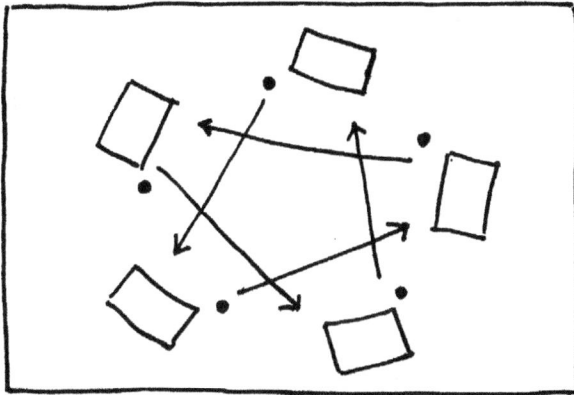

To play:
- Set up five teams identified by their sashes, and five gym mats in a loop, spaced equally apart. Players are only safe on their mats.
- Place a disc with corresponding team colour a few paces to the right of each mat, to represent each land's Prison.
- Each land's target is not the land to their immediate right, but one away from that: Land One chases Land Three,

---

[84] A variation of the Rock Paper Scissors relationship. This game is similar to Three Lands (See Year 4) but this time with Five Lands, and a little twist.

Land Two chases Land Four, Land Three chases Land Five and Land Five chases Land Two.

- Tagged players go to the Prison of their taggers and are saved by teammates taking them by the hand and leading them to their home base. One player may only save one Prisoner at a time. When linked, both players are safe from being tagged.
- Prisoners may form a rescue chain stretching from Prison to their home base, as long as the newest prisoner has at least one foot on the Prison base.

Variations:
- After a while, change directions of the tag: Land One chases Land Four; Land Five chases Land Three; Land Four chases Land Two; Land Three chases Land One. Remember to change coloured discs of Prison to the other side of each land.

2. Doctor Dodge

Equipment: Several soft dodge balls

Skills: Spatial awareness, agility, teamwork, throwing and catching, strategy

Imagery: Two kingdoms are at war and soldiers on both sides are hurling and dodging fireballs, and many get injured. Luckily, one person in each kingdom is a doctor with incredible healing powers. The soldiers do their best to protect their doctor and keep his identity a secret, or risk losing him to enemy fire.

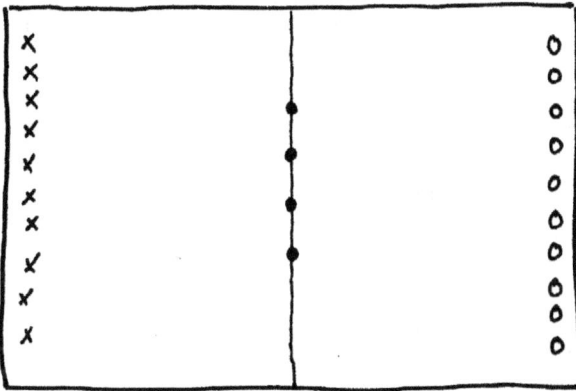

To play:
- Set up two teams and two territories, each team playing from their territory. Each team chooses their Doctor and hides their identity from the other team.
- On the centre line, place several balls. At the signal to start, soldiers from both team rush to gain control of the balls and aim them at their opponents (from the shoulder, waist or knee down).
- Players may dodge a ball but may not catch it.

- A tagged player falls on the spot and waits for the Doctor, who discreetly goes behind him and places his hand on the soldier's back. The healed soldier should not make the rescue obvious but wait for the Doctor to move away before re-joining the game. This can take between 5 -10 seconds.
- If the Doctor is hit, the wounded will no longer be saved.
- The game ends when one team has wounded all the enemy soldiers.

Variations:
- A player may deflect the ball or catch the ball on the full. Here the forearms and hands may be used and not counted towards a tag. If a player catches a ball on the full, the thrower is wounded.
- Game ends when the Doctor is wounded.
- When a Doctor is down, any player who catches a ball on the full is endowed with special healing qualities and has 5 seconds to save as many wounded as possible, including the Doctor.

3. Kings and Queens (1)

Equipment: Coloured sashes for each team, two - six soft dodge balls

Skills: Spatial awareness, agility, teamwork, throwing and catching, strategy

Imagery: Two kingdoms, each lead by a powerful and sorcerous King or Queen, are at war. Captured knights languish in their enemy's dungeon, unless saved by their fellow knights throwing magic fireballs into the dungeon. Knights who catch the ball on the full are magically transported safely back in their territory. If too many of their fellow knights are in the dungeon, the King or Queen may allow themselves to be captured, and then catch a fireball to magically free everyone in the dungeon.

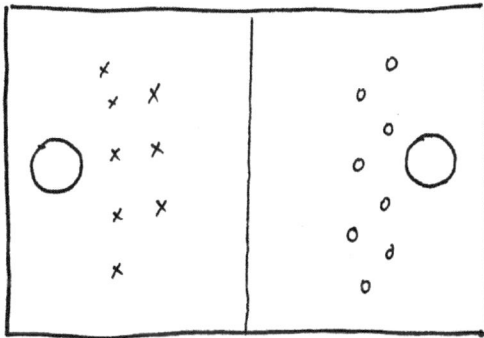

To play:
- Set up two groups and two territories, each group playing from one territory, and may not cross into enemy territory. The aim is to get all their opponents out.
- Each group selects a King or Queen, who is identified with a double sash.
- At the far end of each territory, mark out the Dungeon, a circle big enough for half the class to stand in.

- One person in each team has a small foam ball, and they start the battle at a given signal.
- Each team tries to tag their opponents (shoulders and below) with the ball, and to dodge being tagged.
- Players may protect themselves by deflecting the ball with their forearms (from elbow to hands). They may also catch a ball thrown at them, in which case, the person who threw the ball at them is sent to their opponent's dungeon.
- They may not run when in possession of the ball, but may pivot on the spot, and relay the ball.
- Tagged players go to their opponent's dungeon, and are saved by catching a ball (on the full, without it bouncing) thrown to them by their teammates. Players who catch a ball save themselves, but when a King or Queen catches a ball, they save everyone on their team.
- The game ends when all players of one team are in the dungeon.

Variations:
- Introduce extra balls
- When a prisoner catches a ball on the full, they are free, and are allowed one shot at a defending Knight before leaving the Dungeon. The tagged defender then has to go the opponent's Dungeon.

4. Kings and Queens (2)[85]

Equipment: Coloured sashes for each team, two - six soft dodge balls

Skills: Spatial awareness, agility, teamwork, throwing and catching, strategy

Imagery: Two kingdoms, each lead by a powerful and sorcerous King or Queen, are at war. Each King or Queen directs battle from the rear of the battlefield – their opponent's rear. Injured knights are not battle fit, and are sent to the infirmary, where they continue to support their knights on the sideline. They are healed and may re-join the battle when a teammate in the battle zone catches the enemy's enchanted arrow.

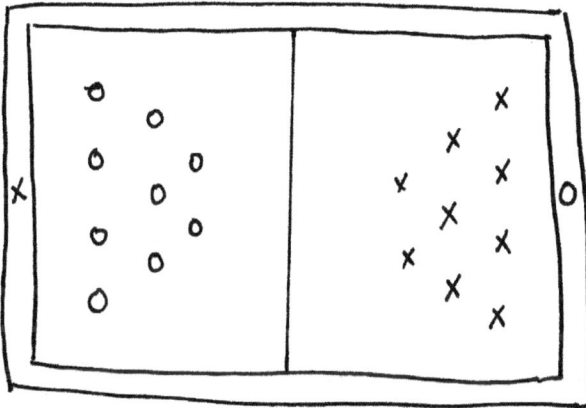

To play:
- Set up two groups and two territories. Each group plays from their territory, and may not cross into enemy territory. The aim is to get all their opponents out.
- Each group selects a King or Queen, who is identified with a double sash.

---

[85] Similar to King and Queens (1) and King Dodge but played with different territory boundaries.

- Each King or Queen stands at the rear of their opponent's territory, just outside the boundary line, with one or more dodge balls. They begin the game by attempting to hit their opponents (shoulders and below) with the ball.
- Players may dodge the ball and protect themselves by deflecting the ball with their forearms (from elbows to hands). They may also catch the ball on the full, thrown at them, in which case the person who threw the ball at them is out. If a King or Queen's throw is caught, they are out of play for a pre-specified time (e.g. one minute).
- Each team tries to tag their opponents (shoulders and below) with the ball. They may pivot on the spot or relay the ball to their teammates, but they may not run when in possession of the ball.
- A tagged player is 'injured' and joins his King or Queen at the far end of the opponent's territory or along the boundaries of the enemy territory. They continue to support the battle by tagging opponents with balls that have strayed out of play, or by balls passed to them from their teammates still in the battle zone.
- If a player catches a ball on the full, they save one teammate who re-joins the game in the battle zone.
- When a team has only one player in the battle zone, the King or Queen enters the battle zone, and together with their last Knight, try to salvage the battle and save their knights.
- The game ends when all the players have been tagged and are off court.

5. Come Hither, Gallant Knights

Equipment: Two to four sets of different coloured sashes

Skills: Spatial awareness, agility, teamwork, throwing and catching

Imagery: Every King or Queen needs loyal Knights to protect and serve the kingdom. So they go to where good soldiers are said to be found and try to persuade them to become their knights before another King or Queen does.

To play:
- Choose one or two Kings and one or two Queens who stand in the middle of the play area, each wearing a different coloured sash and each holding a dodge ball. All others are soldiers and they scatter.
- To start, each monarch throws the ball to tag a soldier (shoulders and below). Soldiers may dodge, but not deflect a ball thrown at them. Tagged soldiers receive the same coloured sash as their monarchs, and they help their monarchs tag other soldiers.
- Players may pivot on the spot or relay the ball to their teammates but may not run when in possession of the ball.
- Continue until all soldiers are knighted, or the last few knights can become the new Kings and Queens.

Variations:
- Once all are knighted, and teams are established, they play Team Dodge (See Class 5). Each team tries to tag out all other teams. Tagged players sit out until their tagger is tagged out. The last team remaining is the winner.

6. Snake Dodge

Equipment: One soft dodge ball

Skills: Spatial awareness, agility, teamwork

Imagery: Once upon a time, there was a giant snake who lived in the caves deep in the rainforest. He slipped between the underworld and the upper world through the cracks and holes in the ground. The villagers living near the cave believed that if they tagged the snake's tail, it would bring them power.

To play:
- Six to seven players form a Snake line within a circle formed by the students. The front of the Snake line is the 'Head', and the last person is the 'Tail'. The Snake line works together to protect its 'Tail' from being tagged.
- One person in the circle begins by throwing the ball to tag the 'Tail' (from knees and below). Players in the circle may relay the ball to each other.
- When the 'Tail' is tagged, he joins the circle and the second last player in the line becomes the new tail.
- The game ends when only one player remains.

Variations:
- Tagger becomes the new Snake Head, and the 'Tail' joins the circle. Game ends after a specified time.

7. Quadrant Dodge

Equipment: Two soft dodge balls, sashes for teams, cone markers, or chalk or rope to mark boundaries

Skills: Spatial awareness, agility, teamwork, throwing and catching

Imagery: Two kingdoms are at war, and have amassed their armies and are facing off for a battle. Each side has taken a stand near the cross junction of the land and are battling for control. Who will win this battle?

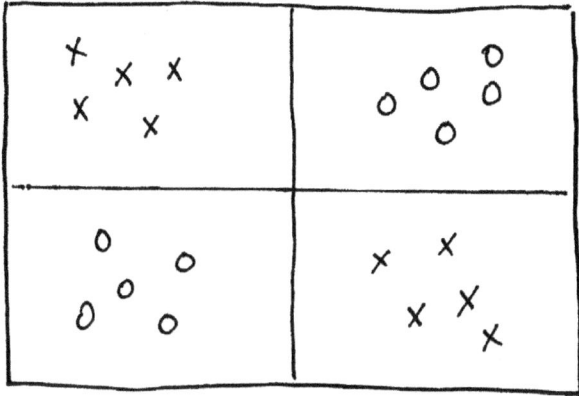

To play:
- Divide the area into four sections or quadrants, and the class into two teams, with one team wearing sashes. Half of each team position themselves in diagonally opposite section. Each team has a ball, and players may move freely within their two quadrants, but not into the other team's territory.
- On the signal to start, each team tries to tag their opponents with the ball, from shoulders and below, and tries to get the whole team out.

- Players may pivot and relay the ball to their teammates, but may not run when in possession of the ball. They may dodge, deflect (from elbows to hands) or catch a ball thrown at them on the full.
- Tagged players are 'injured' and stand outside their quadrants and may retrieve balls for their teams but not take an active part.
- If a player catches an opponent's ball thrown to them on the full, the thrower is out. Each catch also frees one of the catcher's injured teammates who may re-join the game.
- The team that eliminates the other is the winner.

8. Dragon's Lair

Equipment: One hula hoop per person

Skills: Spatial awareness, strategy, agility, teamwork

Imagery: An unfriendly and smelly dragon wanted so much to have his own lair in trendy Dragon Mountain. He could imagine himself curled up in a cave, beside a little fire and a nice cup of hot chocolate. However, none of the other dragons want him in their neighbourhood, so they do their best to foil his house hunting plans.

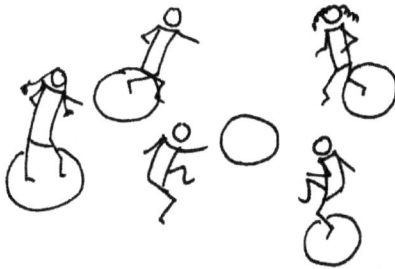

To play:
- Scatter hula hoops (Lairs) around the play area. All are dragons in their lair except one child who is Smelly Dragon without a lair. Leave an empty hoop.
- Smelly Dragon tries to step into the empty hoop, but the others try to prevent this, preferably one close by who can beat it to the empty hoop. Thwarted, Smelly Dragon tries to step into the newly vacated hoop, but someone else needs to quickly step in to prevent this from happening.
- If Smelly manages to step into a hoop, the dragon closest to, or the one who attempted to but failed to thwart Smelly becomes the new Smelly Dragon, and the game continues in the same manner. The game ends after a specified time.

9. Four - Way Storm the Castle[86]

Equipment: Coloured sashes for each team, and six bean bags per team of corresponding team colours (e.g. six blue, six red, six yellow, six green), cones, rope or chalk to mark boundaries

Skills: Spatial awareness, agility, speed, teamwork, throwing and catching

Imagery: A long time ago, Four Lords were each granted a Kingdom to rule. A magic Key was also given to each Lord, which consisted of six interlocking parts. Promising to live in harmony, each Lord entrusted two pieces of their key to each of the three Lords. The Kingdoms lived in harmony for many generations, but in time, greed, jealousy and intolerance ate away at the hearts of men and they started to feud. Now they are vying for control of the land and the title of Emperor! To do so, each Kingdom needs to retrieve all six parts of their Key.

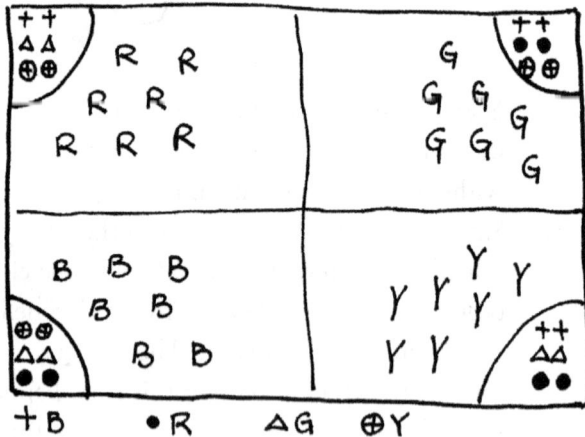

---

[86] A more advanced version of Strom the Castle (1&2), this time with 4 groups.

To play:
- Set up four teams (identified by sashes) and four quadrants. Each group takes one quadrant, which is their safe zone.
- At each corner, mark a place for the Castle.
- Within each castle, place the six keys (six bean bags consisting of two of each team's colours except their own). For example, in Red castle, place two green, two blue and two yellow bean bags. And in Green castle, place two blue, two red and two yellow bean bags, and so on.
- At the signal to start, players attempt to invade the other team's treasury to retrieve their coloured keys and to bring it safely back to their castle without being tagged. So Red invades all other castles to retrieve red keys; Green invades all other castles to retrieve green keys, and so on.
- Players may only retrieve one key at a time.
- Tagged players must surrender any treasure in their possession, bob down on the spot and wait for rescue by team members taking them by their hand and leading them back to their safe zone. They are safe when linked.
- The game ends when one team has retrieved all six pieces of their key.

Variations:
- Tagged players have to go to the tagger's dungeon and await rescue by their teammates.
- Place any number of bean bags within each castle and players attempt to steal as many treasures as possible. The winning team is the one with the highest number of treasures after a specified time.

10. Prisoner's Base

Equipment: Sashes for team, cones or markers for boundaries and zones

Skills: Spatial awareness, agility, strategy and teamwork

Imagery: Prisoners of war are often kept in dark, damp, smelly and rat-infested prisons. It was a most dismal place. Two warring kingdoms have an elite member of their kingdoms imprisoned and are now trying to stage a rescue effort.

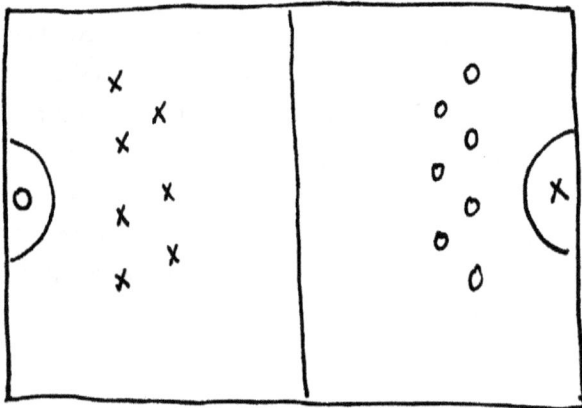

To play:
- Set up two teams and two territories, each team playing from one territory, which is their safe zone. At the end of each territory, mark out a Prison to hold enemy prisoners (large enough for a whole team).
- Each team selects one member to be Prisoner (usually a fast runner) who starts in the enemy's prison.
- At the signal to start, each team attempts a rescue effort. They break into the enemy prison and lead their teammate by their hand, back to home territory, without either being caught, while at the same time, preventing their opponents from doing the same.

- If a team member is caught while attempting a rescue, they join their teammate in Prison and have to wait for rescue.
- If a team member manages to break into prison, they may remain there safely until an opportune moment for both to break out. They do not receive a free walk home, as either can be caught and imprisoned while breaking out.
- The winning team is the one who has captured all their opponents, or the team with the most prisoners after a specified time.

11. Dark Knights

Equipment: Volleyball court or ropes / cones to mark boundary, hula hoops, gym mat, and lots of small dodge balls

Skills: Spatial awareness, agility, ball handling skills, teamwork

Imagery: The Dark Prince has usurped the throne and has exiled his rival, the White King, and imprisoned the King's loyal knights in island fortresses that cannot be easily accessed. However, he has underestimated the loyalty of the remaining White Knights, who are intent on freeing their friends and re-instating their King.

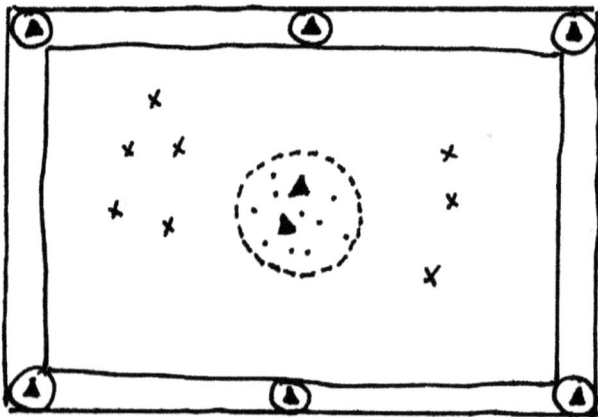

To play:
- Use a volleyball court or set up a play area similar in size with rope, cones etc. Mark out a circle large enough for half the team (or use a gym mat) in the middle and place dodge balls within. Place hula hoops on the outskirts of this boundary as gaols.
- Divide the class into two equal groups, the White Knights and the Dark Knights. Two White Knights begin in the

Circle, and the others imprisoned in hula hoops on the outskirts of the boundary. The defending Dark Knights are scattered about the court.

- The two White Knights begin by throwing the dodge balls to the captured Knights in the hula hoops. If a captured White Knight catches the ball on the full, they are freed and join the other White Knights in the circle to help free the others still imprisoned.
- Dark Knights may not enter the circle and White Knights may only throw the ball from the circle and may only leave the circle to collect stray balls.
- Dark Knights who intercept a ball simply releases the ball on to the court to continue defending.
- Imprisoned Knights may not stray out of their gaol, but may pass on stray balls within their reach.
- The game ends when all the White Knights are freed, or after a specified time.

Variations:
- An imprisoned Knight who catches the ball on the full has 5 seconds during which to tag a Dark Knight (shoulders and below). If tagged, Dark Knights sit out until saved by a team mate who catches a ball on the full.
- If a Dark Knight catches the ball on the full, the thrower is imprisoned.

12. Who will be King?

Equipment: Ten to fifteen skittles

Skills: Skill, agility, balance, strength

Imagery: The land has been plunged into tribal war and chaos. But the soothsayers have prophesised that in its darkest hour, the one true King will rise to unit them all. This King will brave the Great Serpent's pit and survive, and in doing so, will lead the land into a period of peace and prosperity. Great warriors come from afar to test their strength and valour. Who will be crowned King?

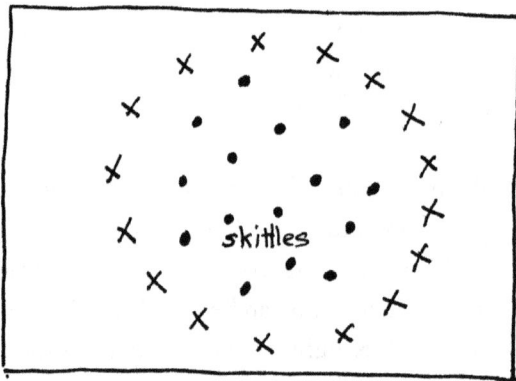

To play:
- All players clasp hands, facing in to encircle the Serpent's Pit, which contains several skittles (poison), placed with space between through which a player might step.
- At the signal to start, players push or pull as hard as they can make others touch or knock over the skittles, taking care to avoid doing the same. Anyone who touches or knocks over the skittles, or unclasps their hands has to leave the circle, the skittles being replaced.

- Those who leave the main circle, form a sub circle with the same objective of evading the poison while attempting to get others poisoned. A player from the sub circle who is poisoned, leaves the second sub circle to form a third sub circle, and so on.
- The last person in the first circle is crowned the King.

Variations:
- When several circles have been formed, the winners of these circles may form a circle at the close of the game to play to determine the final winner.
- Instead of skittles, place one large cone or soft object in the middle. Players who are poisoned, stay out.
- Mark out a square about three to four paces on the ground. Players entering the poison pit sits out. When the circle becomes too small and it is no longer possible for players to stand around the square, the remaining players stand within it. Each player keeps their hands crossed over their chest and tries to push the others out of the square. The last one remaining is crowned King.

13. Run the Gauntlet (Line Dodge)

Equipment: Six to eight soft dodge balls, cones to mark boundary lines, several bean bags or flags as treasures

Skills: Spatial awareness, agility, speed, teamwork, throwing and catching

Imagery: Viking invaders have been sighted marching up to the Castle, and Knights of the kingdom are preparing to battle and defend their Castle. They station their cannons in anticipation, and fire cannonballs at the invaders who try to raid their treasury.

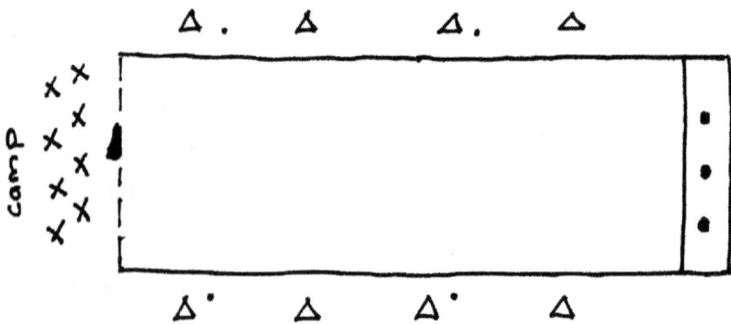

To play:
- Set up two teams, the Vikings and the Defending knights.
- Mark two parallel lines in the centre of the play area about 3 metres apart. At one end of the run is the Viking camp, and at the end of the run is the Treasury where three treasures (bean bags) are placed.
- The Defending Knights position themselves along both sides of the parallel lines, and the Viking invaders start at their camp.
- At the signal to start, the Viking invaders (two at a time) brave the cannon fire (dodge balls) from the Knight

defenders in their attempt to reach the treasures, and to bring it safely back to their camp.

- When Viking invaders are tagged by canon fire (dodge balls), they have to return to Camp and join the end of the line for their turn to invade again. The next invader in line steps in to attempt the raid.

- If a Viking reaches the Treasury, they may remain there and wait for an opportune time to return to camp, but the treasury can only hold four invaders at any time.

- Viking invaders may also be tagged on their return run. If they are in possession of a treasure when tagged by cannon fire, they must surrender the stolen treasures before returning to their camp.

- The game ends when all three treasures have been captured, or after a specified time. Teams then swap roles.

Variations:
- Tagged Vikings may only have one (two or three) tries at raiding the treasury, after which they sit out. The game ends when all Viking invaders are out.

14. Cat and Mouse (7)[87]

Equipment: None

Skills: Agility, strategy, speed, quick reaction

Imagery: Cat and Mouse were once very good friends, but they had a falling out. The Cat accuses the Mouse of being cunning and the Mouse accuses the Cat of being lazy. And now whenever they meet, tensions flare! (For the story, see Cat and Mouse (1)).

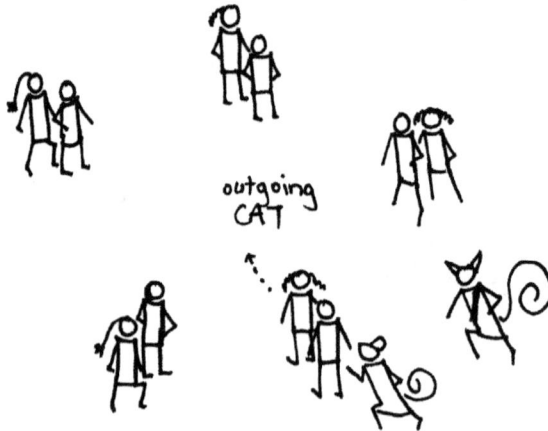

outgoing
CAT

To play:
- One Cat to chase one Mouse. All others are Safe Houses, standing in pairs, one in front of the other, in a circle (or scattered throughout the play area).
- The Mouse has to find a safe house, by standing in front or behind a pair. An incoming Mouse who stands in the front of a pair releases an outgoing Mouse at the rear.

---

[87] Spatial and cognitive demands increase as danger comes in all directions.

- An incoming Mouse who stands at the back, releases a Cat in the front. It alerts the person in front that they are now the new Cat, by tapping on their shoulder.
- If the Mouse is caught, it swaps roles with the Cat.

Variations:
- Standing in pairs side by side. An incoming Mouse standing on the right of a pair releases a Mouse on the left. An incoming Mouse standing on the left of a pair releases a Cat on the right. This variation is more demanding.

15.Cat and Mouse (8)[88]

Equipment: None

Skills: Agility, strategy, speed, quick reaction

Imagery: Cat and Mouse were once very good friends, but they had a falling out. The Cat accuses the Mouse of being cunning and the Mouse accuses the Cat of being lazy. And now whenever they meet, tensions flare! (For the story, see Cat and Mouse (1)).

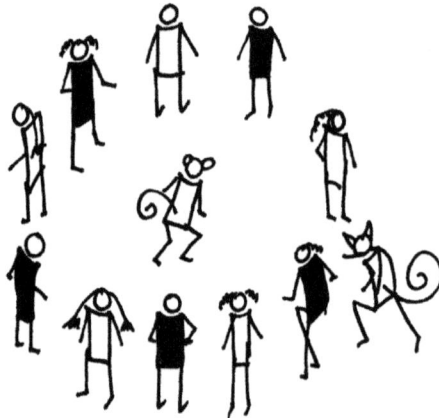

To play:
- One Cat to chase one Mouse. All others are Cats standing in a circle, alternately facing in and out. The Mouse starts inside the circle, and the Cat starts outside, and gives chase.
- The Mouse may step in and out of the circle, but an outside Cat may not enter the circle, and an inside Cat may not exit the circle.
- To catch the Mouse when it is inside the circle, the outside Cat needs to release an inward facing Cat to hunt. It does

---

[88] This version is also spatially demanding and cognitively challenging.

so by tapping the back of an inward facing Cat, the signal to release it to hunt. The incoming Cat then takes over the spot vacated by the outgoing Cat.

- To catch the Mouse while it is outside the circle, the inside Cat needs to release an outward facing Cat, in the same manner above. A tagged Mouse becomes the new Cat and the game continues.

16. Panjandrum[89] (or Body Guard)

Equipment: Three sashes

Skills: Strategy, spatial awareness, teamwork, agility

Imagery: The Grand Panjandrum himself is setting out of his mansion to attend the opening of the grand bazaar. The poor peasants in the street try to touch him for good luck and fortune, so they could be as grand as he is. Can his burly Bodyguards protect him?

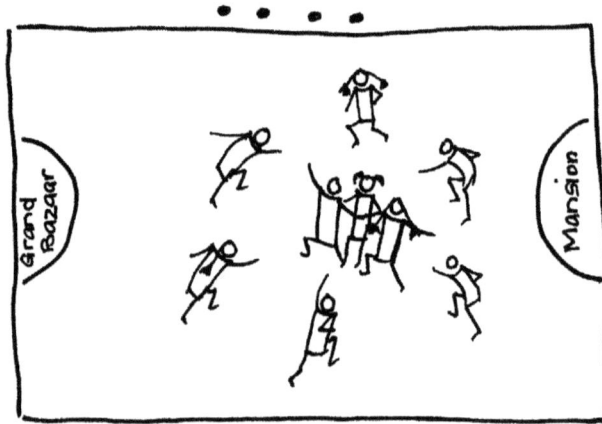

To play:
- Mark off an area at one end of the play area as the Panjandrum's Mansion and an area on the opposite as the Grand Bazaar. Designate another area as the Hospital.
- One player is chosen as the Panjandrum and two players are the Bodyguards. All others are Peasants.

---

[89] A Panjandrum is a powerful personage or pretentious official, a nonsense word coined by British actor and playwright Samuel Foote around 1755. This game is adapted from a game found in (Bancroft, 1909).

- Starting at the mansion, the Bodyguards clasp hands and precede the Panjandrum, shielding him from the peasants, as they make their way to the Grand Bazaar. The guards will shift about their charge to avoid the peasants and the Panjandrum himself may evade them by moving around his guards.
- Tagged peasants are sent to hospital. There are only four hospital beds and when the fifth one comes, the first one is discharged.
- If the Panjandrum and his guards make it to the Grand Bazaar, they have won and a new trio is chosen.
- If a peasant manages to tag the Panjandrum, they swap places and new Guards are chosen and the game goes on as before.

17. Everyman in his own Den[90]

Equipment: None

Skills: Strategy, spatial awareness, teamwork, agility

Imagery: Once upon a time a wise leader gave his sons an arrow each and told them to break it, which they did easily. Then he gave them a bunch of arrows and told them to do the same, which they could not. He told them that strength lies in unity!

To play:
- Each player selects a Den (safe place) for himself (along the wall, corners of the room, etc.)
- Any player may start by running out from his den. A second player runs out and tries to tag him, while a third may tag either of the two, and so on. The objective is to make captives of others before you and avoid being captured by those after you.
- Players may return to their den at any time, and on venturing forth again, has the advantage of being able to capture any before him.
- Any player caught joins his captor in his den and as one, they venture out to tag others. If either is caught, they both join their captors. One player may capture one opponent at a time.
- Players gradually gather into groups and the group that captures all the players is the winner.

Variations:
- The group with the most players after a specified time wins.

---

[90] Game adapted from (Bancroft, 1909), also known as Dare Base.

18. On your Head be it! (Three Bounce)

Equipment: One soft dodge ball, cones or lines on the ground to mark boundary or ideally, a small, enclosed area with walls to mark boundaries

Skills: Speed, agility, ball handling, strategy, spatial awareness

Imagery: The Celts believed that severed heads could continue to live, eat, talk and sing independently of the body, and that the more powerful the individual, the more powerful the severed head's ability to have healing properties and foretell the future. That is why many severed heads are placed near wells and springs to make the water sacred. Now, this particular head was lonely being stuck in the damp well, so he told the villagers that he needed fresh air three hours every month, and that they needed to keep his head aloft and not let it touch the ground. Any villager who drops his head is punished by doing sentry duty to guard the well and the village.

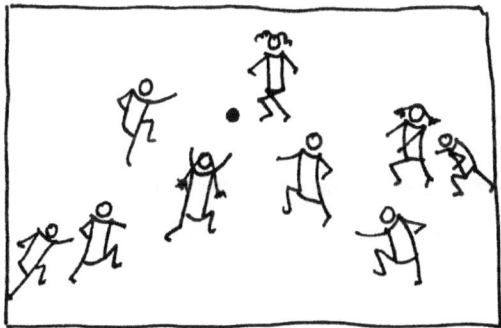

To play:
- Set up a play area with very clear boundaries (e.g. with lines, cones, rope or walls).
- All players are Villagers whose main objective is to keep the Severed Head (ball) in the air without letting it touch the ground.

- The teacher begins by tossing the Severed Head (ball) into the air, and Villagers scramble to keep it from touching the ground.
- Up to two bounces are allowed, but on the third bounce, the Villager closest to the ball is caught out.
- Villagers caught out have to do sentry duty, by going to any part of the boundary line and making contact with it (one foot on the rope or line, or one hand on the wall). They may move along the boundary as long as they maintain some form of contact with it.
- Villagers on the boundary may not touch the ball. They are able to re-join the game when they tag an unwary Villager still in the game, who comes too close. Tagger then swap places with the tagged.
- Methods of keeping the ball off the ground include bumping it with palms, fists or forearms (like in volleyball) or hitting or bouncing it (like in basketball) so that it bounces up.
- Villagers may not touch the ball twice in a row.
- The game ends when there is one Villager left in the game, or after a specified time.

Variations:
- Have a second ball. The villagers invite the severed head of the Norse God, Mimir, for a consult.
- Apply the 'Decimate'[91] rule, where the teacher randomly counts and selects the 10th person to be sent out. Players sent out may only re-join the game by tagging an unwary villager still in the game.

---

[91] 'Decimate' was a Roman military discipline action in which the 10th person in a group was executed. This variation was inspired by a conversation with a dear friend and colleague, Joanne Mills.

Appendix: Verses and Songs

1. **Rat-a-tat**
   Rat-a-tat, rat-a-tat,
   Who can it be?
   Rat-a-tat, rat-a-tat,
   Let's go and see!
   There is a postman
   Knocking at the door,
   Have you any letters?
   One, two, three, four, five!
   One, two, three, four, five!

   (nursery rhyme)

2. **Sally Goes Round the Sun**
   Sally goes round the sun
   Sally goes round the moon
   Sally goes round the chimney pot
   On a Saturday afternoon.

   (nursery rhyme)

3. **Incy Wincy Spider**
   Incy Wincy Spider
   Climbed up the waterspout
   Down came the rain and washed poor Incy out
   Up came the sun and dried up all the rain
   So Incy Wincy spider climbed up the spout again.

   (nursery rhyme)

4. **The Glow-worm**
   Oh, I wish I were a glow worm,
   for a glow worm's never glum,
   'cause how can you be grumpy
   when the sun shines out your bum?

   (author unknown)

5. **Where is Thumbkin?**
   Where is Thumbkin? Where is Thumbkin?
   Here I am. Here I am.
   How are you today sir? Very well I thank you.
   Run away. Run away.

   (nursery rhyme)

   (Set to the tune of "Are you sleeping, Brother John".

6. **Slowly, Slowly Creeps the Snail**
   Slowly, slowly, very slowly
   Creeps the garden snail
   Slowly, slowly, very slowly
   Up the garden rail
   Slowly, slowly very slowly
   creeps the garden snail
   Slowly, slowly, very slowly,
   Down the garden rail.

   (nursery rhyme)

7. **Hickety Pickety, My Black Hen**
   Hickety, Pickety, my black hen,
   She lays eggs for gentlemen;
   Gentlemen come every day
   To see what my black hen doth lay,
   Sometimes nine and sometimes ten,
   Hickety Pickety, my black hen.

   (nursery rhyme)

8. **Moses Supposes**
   Moses supposes his toe-ses were roses
   But Moses supposes erroneously
   For nobody's toe-ses are posies of roses
   As Moses supposes his toe-ses to be.

   (tongue twister)

9. **One Two Buckle My Shoe**
   One, two, buckle my shoe
   Three, four, knock at the door
   Five, six, pick up sticks
   Seven, eight, lay them straight
   Nine, ten, a big fat hen
   Eleven, twelve, dig and delve
   Thirteen, fourteen, maids a-courting
   Fifteen, sixteen, maids in the kitchen
   Seventeen, eighteen, maids in waiting
   Nineteen, twenty, my plate's empty.

   (nursery rhyme)

10. **Whether the Weather**
    Whether the weather be fine
    Or whether the weather be not
    Whether the weather be cold
    Or whether the weather be hot
    We'll weather the weather
    Whatever the weather
    Whether we like it or not.

    (tongue twister)

11. **Woodchuck**

    How much wood would a woodchuck chuck, if a woodchuck could chuck wood?

    A woodchuck would chuck all he could, if a woodchuck could chuck wood.

    (tongue twister)

12. **Peter Piper**

    Peter Piper picked a peck of pickled peppers
    A peck of pickled peppers Peter Piper picked
    If Peter Piper picked a peck of pickled peppers
    Where's the peck of pickled peppers Peter Piper picked?

    (tongue twister)

13. **Betty Botter**

    Betty Botter bought a bit of butter
    But the bit of butter Betty Botter bought was bitter
    So Betty Botter bought a better bit of butter
    To make her bitter butter better.

    (tongue twister)

14. **I had a Little Nut Tree**

    I had a little nut tree
    Nothing would it bear
    But a silver nutmeg

    And a golden pear
    The King of Spain's daughter
    Came to visit me,
    And all for the sake
    Of my little nut tree.

    (tongue twister)

15. **The Queen of Hearts**
    The Queen of Hearts,
    She made some tarts,
    All on a summer's day;
    The Knave of Hearts,
    He stole those tarts,
    And took them clean away.

    The King of Hearts
    Called for the tarts,
    And beat the Knave full sore;
    The Knave of Hearts
    Brought back the tarts,
    And vowed he'd steal no more.

    (tongue twister)

16. **She Sells Sea Shells**
    She sells sea shells by the seashore
    The shells she sells by the seashore are sea shells for sure.

    (tongue twister)

17. **Brave and True I Will Be**
    Brave and true will I be,
    Each good deed sets me free,
    Each kind word makes me strong.
    I will fight for the right!
    I will conquer the wrong!

    —Rudolf Steiner

18. **The Spider and the Fly**
  "Will you walk into my parlour?" said the Spider to the Fly,
  "Tis the prettiest little parlour that ever you did spy;
  The way into my parlour is up a winding stair,
  And I have many curious things to show you when you are there."
  "Oh no, no," said the Fly, "to ask me is in vain;
  For who goes up your winding stair can ne'er come down again."
          —Mary Howitt

Bibliography

Ayres, A. J. (2007). *Sensory integration and the Child: Understandinng Hidden Sensory Challenges.* USA: Western Psychological Services.

Ballard, C. (2020, January 8). *Are Kids' Sports Becoming Too Competitive?* Retrieved from Experience Life: https://experiencelife.com/article/putting-kids-and-fun-back-into-kids-sports/

Bancroft, J. (2008, May 31). *Games for the Playground, Home, School and Gymnasium.* Retrieved from Project Gutenberg: http://www.gutenberg.org/ebooks/25660

Banks, D. (2016, Apr 5). *What is brain plasticity and why is it so important?* Retrieved October 9, 2020, from The Conversation: https://theconversation.com/what-is-brain-plasticity-and-why-is-it-so-important-55967

Brooking-Payne, K. (1998). *Games Children Play: How games and sport help children develop.* Hawthorn Press.

Bruegel, P. (1564). *Kunsthistorisches_Museum.* Retrieved January 20, 2021, from https://www.insidebruegel.net/#p/v=udroom&lan=en&a=1017&x=s:3_l:1_v1:1017,vis,41518.5,29943.5,0.00714

Burke, S. (2010). *Lighting the Literacy Fire.* Littleleaves Press.

Cheatum, B. a. (2000). *Physical Activities for Improving Children's Learning and Behaviour.* USA: Human Kinetics.

Cohut, M. (2109, September 12). *Study of foot painters adds to evidence of brain's adaptability.* Retrieved from Medical News Today: https://www.medicalnewstoday.com/articles/326321

Cunningham, J. (2004). *Working with Curriculum in Australian Rudolf Steiner Schools.* NSW: Rudolf Steiner Schools of Australia, an Association.

Dascy, E. (1930, September 20). *The Sydney Morning Herald.* Retrieved January 7, 2021, from Trove: https://trove.nla.gov.au/newspaper/article/16695986

Dendtler, C. (2018, August 25). *The Eight-Year-Old: A View From Waldorf Education*. Retrieved December 26, 2020, from The Parenting Passageway: https://theparentingpassageway.com/category/development/age-eight/

Down, R. (2012, January 10). *The Role of the Teacher-Artist in the Seven Fold Waldorf School*. Retrieved January 4, 2021, from The Online Waldorf Library: https://www.waldorflibrary.org/articles/604-the-role-of-the-teacher-artist-in-the-seven-fold-waldorf-school

Dr Geier, D. (2020, September 14). *Examining the effects of sport specialization on mental health of young athletes*. Retrieved from The Post and Courier: https://www.postandcourier.com/sports/examining-the-effects-of-sport-specialization-on-mental-health-of-young-athletes/article_ec9872b2-e9e9-11e9-a76f-2f3a79047141.html

Dr White, R. (2012). *The Power of Play: A Research Summary of Play and Learning*. Minnesota, USA: Minnesota Children's Museum.

Freeman, D. (n.d.). Lecture notes and personal communication.

Gilb, S. S. (1962). *The Glib Revised Card File of Games*. Lexington, Kentucky: Hurst Printing Company.

Goddard, S. (2002). *Reflexes, Learning and Behaviour: A Window Into the Child's Mind*. USE: Fern Ridge Press.

Greenaway, K. (1889 reprinted 1986). *Book of Games*. Hong Kong: Chancellor Press London.

Hannaford, C. (2011). *The Dominance Factor: How Knowing Your Dominant Eye, Ear, Brain, Hand and Foot Can Improve Your Learning*. Utah, USA: Great River Books.

Hartman, P. C. (2013, June). *Loving Authority and Discipline*. Retrieved December 26, 2020, from Rudolf Steiner Centre, Toronto: https://www.rsct.ca/blog?blogid=12678&&modex=blogid&modexval=12678

Holecko, C. (2020, December 3). *When Should Kids Start Playing Competitive Sports?* Retrieved from Very Well Family: https://www.verywellfamily.com/when-should-kids-start-competitive-sports-1257040

Hungerford, T. (n.d.). *Games with Tom*. Melbourne Rudolf Steiner School Training Seminar.

Jensen, E. (2005). *Teaching with the Brain in Mind*. USA: Association for Supervision and Curriculum Develpment.

Johnson, G. E. (1907 reprinted 2015). *Education by Plays and Games*. Ginn and Company (Leopold Classic Library).

Kent Community Health NHS Foundation Trust. (n.d.). *BEAM Education and Movement Programme*. Kent Community Health NHS Foundation Trust.

Kischnick, R. (1979). *Games, Gymnastics, Sport in Child Development*. Rudolf Steiner Press.

Kornberger, H. (2013). *The Power of Stories: Nurturing Children's Imagination and Consciousness*. Poland: Floris Books.

Krog, D. S. (2010). *Movement Programmes as a means to Learning Readiness*. University of South Africa.

Lackner, A. (2016). *The Life Sense*. Retrieved January 20, 2021, from The Online Waldorf Library: https://www.waldorflibrary.org/images/stories/ Journal_Articles/gw_71lackner2.pdf

Landry, L. a. (1993). *Ready to use P.E. Activities for Grades 5-6*. USA: Parker Publishing Company.

Maffulli, N. (2000, June). *At what age should a child begin regular continuous exercise at moderate or high intensity?* Retrieved from The Western journal of medicine, 172(6), 413.: https://doi.org/10.1136/ewjm.172.6.413

Mark, J. J. (2018, May 4). *Augustus*. Retrieved from Ancient History Encyclopedia: https://www.ancient.eu/augustus/

McAllen, A. (1999). *The Extra Lesson*. Fair Oalks,California: Rudolf Steiner College Press.

McMillan, J. a. (2019, January). *Play, Games, and Sports in Childhood – The Right Thing at the Right Time*. Retrieved from Waldorf Today: https://www.waldorftoday.com/2019/01/ play-games-and-sports-in-childhood-the-right-thing-at-the-right-time/

Myers, T. W. (2014). *Anatomy Trains: Mysfacial Meridians for Manual and Movement Therapists*. China: Churchill Lovingstone Elsevier.

Nash-Wortham, M. a. (2000). *Take Time: Movement exercises for parents, teachers and therapists of children with difficulties in speaking, reading, writing and spelling*. England: The Robinswood Press.

Nielsen, D. T. (December 6, 2010). Imagination is as important as facts. *Canberra Times.*

Playground Professional. (2015, March 30). *Movement and Learning: What's the Connection?* Retrieved October 9, 2020, from https://www.playgroundprofessionals.com/play/health-and-safety/movement-and-learning-whats-connection

Rawson, M. &. (2008). *The Education Tasks and Content of the Steiner Curriculum.* East Sussex: Steiner Waldorf Schools Fellowship.

Roh, C.-P. (2012). *The I and the Body in Sensory Existence.* Retrieved October 12, 2020, from Waldorf Library: https://waldorflibrary.org/omages/stories/Journal_Articles/gw63_roh.pdf

Schoorel, E. (2004). *The First Seven Years: Phsiology of Childhood.* CA, USA: Rudolf Steiner College Press.

Soesman, A. (1990). *Out Twelve Senses: Wellsprings of the Soul.* Stroud, UK: Hawthorn Press.

Squareman, C. (1916). *My Book of Indoor Games.* http://www.gutenberg.org/cache/epub/13022/pg13022.txt.

Steiner, R. (1916, June 20). *Toward Imagination: Lecture 3: The Twelve Human Senses.* Retrieved October 14, 2020, from Rudolf Steiner Archive: https://wn.rsachive.org/GA/GA0169/19160620p01.html

Steiner, R. (1923, August 10). *Education: Walking Speaking Thinking (Lecture: S-5382).* Retrieved from Rudolf Steiner Archive and E-Library: https://wn.rsarchive.org/Education/GA307/English/RSPC1943/19230810p01.html

Wil van haren and Rudolf Kischnick, t. b. (1999). *Child's Play 1 and 2.* Hawthorn Press.

Witsenburg, T. (2021, February 5). Personal communication. (A. d. Souza, Interviewer)

World Health Organisation. (2002, April 4). *Physical inactivity a leading cause of disease and disability, warns WHO.* Retrieved October 9, 2020, from World Health Organisation: https://www.who.int/mediacentre/news/releases/release23/en/

About the Author

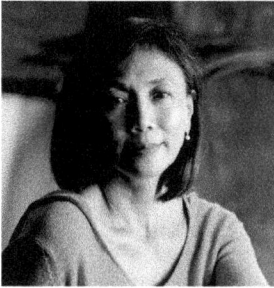

Photo by
Mark.quinstreetpho-
tography@gmail.com

Agnes de Souza is a movement teacher and facilitator, fascinated by the healing effects of movement and bodywork.

A former psychologist in the Air Force, Agnes understands the importance of spatial awareness, psychomotor skills, and quick reaction time, all part of the skillset of a pilot. She traded her suit for motherhood, entered the world of movement and sensory integration and discovered the joys of working with children. She undertook anthroposophical studies, trained in Extra Lesson®, and worked one on one with children with learning difficulties.

Resonating with the therapeutic qualities of Bothmer® Gymnastics and games, Agnes travelled extensively to train for the next ten years, often with her young child in tow, juggling motherhood, obtaining her teaching certification and teaching in a Steiner School. Integrating her experience has resulted in her unique approach to movement education.

Agnes lives in Fremantle, Western Australia, and continues to explore various forms of movement and bodywork. She is trained in Esalen® Massage, aquatic bodywork and yoga, and loves to play games with children and to inspire adults in the craft of movement and games. She is available to facilitate workshops for children, teachers or teachers in training.

Visit Agnes online at www.movementthatmatters.com.au.

www.ingramcontent.com/pod-product-compliance
Lightning Source LLC
Chambersburg PA
CBHW072059020426
42334CB00017B/1563